MW00513254

Ketogenic Air Fryer Cookbook

2 books in 1: The most wanted cookbook to enjoy fried food, save money and time with mouth-watering recipes, from beginners to advanced

James Ball

Legal & Disclaimer

TABLE OF CONTENTS

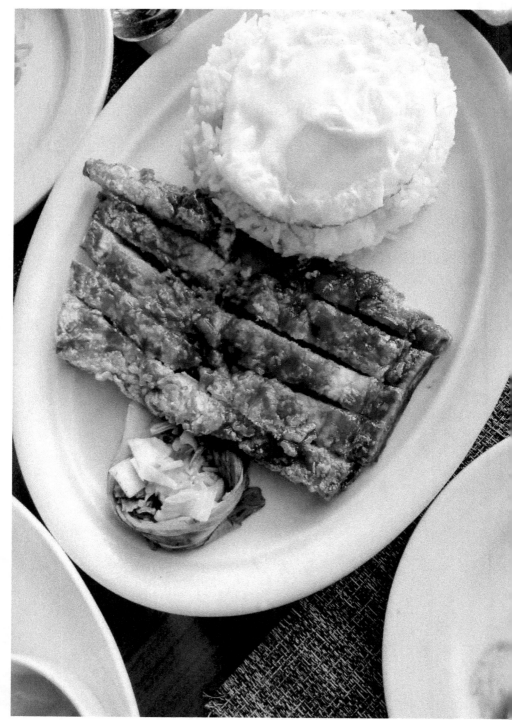

INTRODUCTION

The new air fryer is one of the most versatile cooking appliances on the market today. You will never have to buy another air fryer, which will help you cut your costs and save money. The lid of the Instant Fryer features Instant Clear Technology. It makes your food crispy on the outside and perforated on the inside, which also gives your food a nice brown texture. The lid of the Instant Air Canister Fryer fries the food with much less oil. If you are one of those people who love to deep fry but are also watching out for extra calories, then this kitchen appliance is for you. With just a tablespoon of oil, your fries will be crispy on the outside and tender on the inside.

The Instant Pot is not a new appliance for most people. Your food should taste tempting and not always be unhealthy. Now it's time for the new Instant Pot revolutions to deep fry. This wonderful appliance combines science and art to give you healthy meals for your whole family.

Minimizes unhealthy fats, including trans fats and saturated fats, while preserving important nutrients Instant Pot Air Fryer Crisp comes with many new options for steam, pressure, slow cooker, sous vide, fry, fries, and chicken. In this special book, discover the secret to fast, healthy, and delicious meals with this new kitchen appliance. This book includes a detailed introduction to learn all about this new invention.

This is a complete book with a collection of recipes (appetizers, snacks, poultry, pork, beef, lamb, fish, seafood, vegetables and dessert) that you can effortlessly prepare with the wonderful Instant Pot Air Fryer Crisp. Each recipe is tested to perfection with easy instructions for beginners. Even if you are a first time cook, you can easily prepare all the recipes with simple instructions. Get ready for amazing dishes of crispy, crunchy and caramelized food. Let's find out what this new Instant Pot can do for you.

he Perks of Using the Duo Crisp Air Fryer

There are a lot of perks and benefits of using this appliance in your kitchen. Convenience, diversity, ease of use, tasty, and healthy food are only some benefits that scratch the surface. Let's know something more about how you can benefit from it.

The duality of functions facilitated by this device is something to be proud of. And looking at the control panel, you will get to know the broad scope of features that this device can perform with ease. I have been using two different appliances for pressure cooking and air frying. And let me tell you something that not even the individual appliances can perform these many functions as you are getting with this one.

Just swap the lid:

Turning your pressure cooker into an air fryer is only as hard as changing the lid. And if you would look at it, this changing of the lid transforms everything in your appliance. And to top that, you are well shielded from making any kind of mistake of mixing up the functions. Because you cannot operate the pressure cooker with the air fryer lid resting on the top of the appliance. And the same goes for when you are using it as a pressure cooker.

Placing the Lid:

The Air Fryer and Pressure cooker lid are easily locked in their place without obstructing the power cord outlet given on the appliance. The design is made to be simple and effective. And this is the case with every other Instant Pot appliance, they provide a safe and secure placement. Added to this, you will also get a separate tray to put the air fryer lid after use.

Easy to use Control Panel:

In other devices that have the same functionality or even the other Instant Pot appliances have preset functions. This literally confuses many users. But the Crisp Duo and Air Fryer do not have any such buttons to confuse you. It has just the primary function buttons provided on the front side of the pot. This time they have removed the buttons from the air fryer lid, too, and that is also something that I like about it.

Smart Accessories for a Smart Device:

Different accessories come as an add on with the Air Fryer Crisp Duo. For instance, the trivet that is made to place the food or even the pot after preparations are complete. Or, the double-layered air fryer basket is also something to be proud of with your appliance. Moreover, the multi-level air fryer basket, boiling or dehydrating tray, and the protective pad are some other essential accessories for this appliance.

One-Click Smart Functions:

Although there are no preset buttons on the appliance, you can work with some smart programs. For instance, the "Keep warm," or even the delay start button, adds another level of accessibility to the appliance.

Status Messages to your Rescue:

For a newbie, who is making their maiden attempt at cooking with the instant pot, there are status messages to help them understand their next steps. Messages like Lid, On, Off, Hot,

End, Food, and Burn indicate either the completion of a process or instruct you to take some action while cooking.

All the more, this book is best for those who are looking to start cooking for the first time with such a multi-tasking appliance. You will find information about what all you can do with this appliance along with how to use it best.

Functions of Instant Pot

The control panel of the Air fryer 11-in-1 Air Fryer/Electric Pressure Cooker is very easy to read and comprehend. Though the LED is small, the displays are easy to read, and interface navigation between the functions are relatively simple. Let us look at some quick highlights of the control panel that can help you understand the device better:

The time format on the control panel displays hours on the left and minutes on the right of the colon. Once the timer hits below 1 minute, the right side of the colon indicates the seconds remaining to complete the cooking.

Once the timer goes off, you will automatically see the light on the KEEP WARM button that will keep your food warm until you are back to check the cooker.

The control panel has no pre-sets; however, if you cook a specific dish multiple times, you can add it as a favorite pre-set to have the same function and settings every time you cook that meal.

On the control panel, you will see a button for DELAY START, which you can use if you want to cook a little later. It will ensure that the dish only cooks when you hit the START button, and until then, the panel will save your settings.

In case, if you want to cancel the meal preparation or wish to add or remove anything from the dish, you can always select the CANCEL button on the control panel, and the Instant Pot will immediately stop the cooking procedure.

The left side of the display is for the temperature setting. You can adjust the temperature by using the plus or the minus button.

On the right side of the display is for the timer. With the help of the plus and the minus button, you can change the timer setting.

The LED is a small black screen that appears on the control panel with blue scripts that signifies the settings you are using and also alerts if any of the devices/functions are missing in the Instant Pot.

Features and Specification

Functional Advantages and Applications:

Air Fryer: In this mode, you will have to use the crisp lid, instead of the pressure cooker lid. The function helps in frying the meals depending upon the temperature and time requirement. You can select the temperature after pressing on

AIR FRY,' and set/change the temperature and the time that you wish to cook and then press to START for beginning the cooking.

Default temperature: 400°F / 204°C

Temperature range: 180°F: 400°F / 82°C: 204°C

Suggested use: Fresh / Frozen fries, chicken wings or shrimps

Default cooking time: 00:18

Cooking time range: 00:01: 01:00

Roast: In this function, there is no pre-set, you can choose the temperature, and the time you require to roast your meal or dish and press START to begin the cooking process. Once you have maintained the temperature and the time, the Instant Pot will remember the pre-set in case if you wish to cook the same dish again.

Default temperature: 380°F / 193°C

Temperature range: 180°F: 400°F / 82°C: 204°C

Suggested use: Beef, Lamb, Pork, Poultry, Vegetables, Scalloped potatoes & more

Default cooking time: 00:40

Cooking time range: 00:01: 01:00

Bake: Using the air fryer lid, you can bake any dish that you want. The function remains the same, choose the temperature and the time and hit START to begin the baking process. Make sure to have the lid over the launching or cooling pad when you have finished the baking.

Default temperature: 365°F / 185°C

Temperature range: 180°F: 400°F / 82°C: 204°C

Suggested use: Fluffy and light cakes, pastries, and buns.

Default cooking time: 00:30

Cooking time range: 00:01: 01:00

Broil: In the BROIL option, the appliance comes with a 400°F default temperature setting, which you cannot change. Since it's a broiling option and it is the hottest setting, you can only change the time. Only after pressing the START option, the cooking will begin.

Default temperature: 400°F / 204°C

Temperature range: Not adjustable

Suggested use: Nachos, Onion Soup, Malt cheese, etc.

Default cooking time: 00:08

Cooking time range: 00:01: 00:40

De-hydrate: Just like any other pre-set, this one is also changeable, where you can change the temperature and timer as needed before you begin the process to DE-HYDRATE the meal.

Default temperature: 125°F / 52°C

Temperature range: 105°F: 165°F / 41°C: 74°C

Suggested use: Fruit leather, jerky, dried vegetables etc.

Default cooking time: 07:00

Cooking time range: 01:00: 72:00

Pressure cook: In this setting, it doesn't allow you to choose the temperature as the built-in option available are the frequencies of HIGH and LOW. By clicking on the pressure cook button, you can select the frequency, choose the time for the meal preparation, and hit START. Ensure to change the lid to the pressure cooker lid; otherwise, the control panel will refuse to begin the process.

Pressure level: LO (low: 8 to 2 psi) / HI (high: 12 to 16 psi)

Suggested use: LO: Fish and seafood, Soft vegetables, rice. HI: Eggs, meat, poultry, roots, hard vegetables, oats, beans, grains, bone broth, chili.

Default cooking time: LO: 00:35 / HI: 00:30

Cooking time range: 00:00: 04:00

Sauté: Under this function, it provides high or low-frequency operation and timer control. To begin the sauté, select the settings and press START.

Temperature level: LO (low) / HI (high)

Suggested use: LO: simmer, reduce, thicken, and caramelize. HI: pan sear, stir fry, sauté & brown.

Default cooking time: 00:30

Cooking time range: 00:01: 00:30

Slow Cook: The function is useful when you wish to slow cook the dishes. The timer of this function can go beyond 24 hours as per the recipe requirement, and the frequencies provided shall be either high or low as per the cooking requirements.

Temperature level: LO (low) / HI (high)

Suggested use: LO: All day cooking can set for 6 hours for the best results. HI: faster slow cooking.

Default cooking time: 06:00

Cooking time range: 00:30: 24:00

Steam: It is an ideal option when you wish to steam your dish like rice or dumplings, etc. The pre-set continues to remain the same with the frequency of high or low, and the timer can decide the steaming requirement.

Sous Vide: It is an ideal method for cooking the dish in the Instant Pot for non-fry cooking, which is especially useful for vacuum-sealed food cooking at a precise temperature for an extended period.

Default temperature: 56°C / 133°F

Default cooking time: 03:00

Cooking time range: 00:30: 99:30

Safety features built within the Instant Pot

When the pressure cooker is fully pressurized, you cannot open the lid until and unless the pressure is released. This feature has been incorporated to protect you from harm or damage due to an abrupt release of the lid forcefully.

Another good thing is that you cannot start cooking if the lid is not locked in its set place. Added to it, you will see a message "Lid" being displayed on the control panel.

There is a smart safety function that won't let the temperature go beyond a limit. These limitations are further set as per the program you have opted for preparing the dish.

The food items may get stuck at the bottom, or there is not enough liquid in the pot for the pressure cooker. In that case, there is overheating. To prevent any kind of damage, there is an overheating protection sequence that limits the formation of excessive heat.

The Instant Pot has an automatic pressure control system which maintains the pressure and suspends heating if the pressure inside the pot is more than the desired level.

There are features, specifications, and an introduction to the significant aspects of this book that you would want to know about. Other than this, you will get to read around 80 recipes that you can prepare with this appliance. Some of these recipes can be prepared with the pressure cooker and others with the air fryer. All of them are divided into different meal courses and kinds to help further you decide what you can eat for the morning breakfast, or evening snacks, or even for dinner.

Control Panel

The Instant Pot Crispy Air Fryer Lid is an attachment to the Air fryer Pressure Cooker. Simply put, the New Air fryer + Air Fryer combines air frying with the rest of cooking features with just a swapping of lids. While the pressure cooker lid offers the following functions:

Pressure cook

Sauté

Slow cook

Sous vide

Food warming

On the other hand, the Air fryer lid offers the following:

Air fry

Roast

Bake

Broil

Dehydrate

With its built-in smart programs, Instant Pot makes it easy for everyone to enjoy cooking whether they are chef or novice. Everyone can prepare their favorite healthy meal quick and fast.

FAQ about the Duo Crisp Air Fryer

What is the inner pot made of?

It is primarily made from 304 (18/8) stainless steel with the aluminum core at the 3-ply bottom for optimal use but ensures you that no aluminum comes in contact with the food you're cooking. There is also no aluminum coating and so the inner pot is in compliant with the FDA for safety standard requirements.

The steam rack is likewise made from food grade 304 (18/8) stainless steel, also ensuring safety for the food you're cooking.

The air fryer comes with a ceramic nonstick coating making food easy to remove and the air fryer basket easy to clean.

Can the setting be adjusted when you have started cooking?

Even when you have started cooking, you can still make some adjustments to the cooking time, cooking temperature, and pressure level.

How many appliances can the Air fryer + Air Fryer cover?

With the Air fryer + Instant Pot, you can have your traditional pressure cooker, steamer, slow cooker, food warmer, and sauté pan all in one kitchen device. Added to these, you can also make use of it as an air fryer, broiler, mini-oven, food dehydrator, and broiler.

Are there foods I should avoid putting into the Instant Pot?

Foods that are high in sugar content ay trigger the Instant Pot to give out a burn alert. Also, extra caution is highly recommended when cooking food like applesauce, oatmeal, pearl barley, and noodles that tend to froth, splatter, or foam as they can cause clogging. When preparing these types of foods, make sure not to fill it beyond the 1/2 line as indicated in the inner pot.

To ensure longevity, regular cleaning of the lids and all their parts are important for proper functioning.

Can I use accessories from other brands with my Air fryer + Air Fryer?

It is recommended that you purchase accessories and other spare parts only from stores authorized by Instant Pot Brands Inc. to ensure the highest level of safety.

1. Fish with Capers & Herb Sauce

Basic Recipe

Preparation Time: 5 minutes

Cooking Time: 15 minutes

Servings: 4

Ingredients:

- 2 cod fillets
- ¼ cup almond flour
- 1 teaspoon Dijon Mustard
- 1 egg
- Sauce:
- 2 tablespoons of light sour cream
- 2 teaspoons capers
- 1 tablespoon tarragon, chopped
- 1 tablespoon fresh dill, chopped
- 2 tablespoons red onion, chopped
- 2 tablespoons dill pickle, chopped

Directions:

1. Add all of the sauce ingredients into a small mixing bowl and mix until well blended then place in the fridge.
2. In a bowl mix Dijon mustard and egg and sprinkle the flour over a plate.
3. Dip the cod fillets first into the egg and coat, and then dip them into the flour, coating them on both sides.
4. Preheat your air fryer to 300-degreeFahrenheit, place fillets into air fryer and cook for 10-minutes.
5. Place fillets on serving dishes and Drizzle with sauce and serve.

Nutrition: Calories 198 Fat 9.4g Carbs 17.6g Protein 11g

2. Lemon Halibut

Basic Recipe

Preparation Time: 5 minutes

Cooking Time: 20 minutes

Servings: 4

Ingredients:

- 4 halibut fillets
- 1 egg, beaten
- 1 lemon, sliced
- Salt and pepper to taste
- 1 tablespoon parsley, chopped

Directions:

1. Sprinkle the lemon juice over the halibut fillets.
2. In a food processor mix the lemon slices, salt, pepper, and parsley.
3. Take fillets and coat them with this mixture; then dip fillets into beaten egg.
4. Cook fillets in your air fryer at 350-degreeFahrenheit for 15-minutes

Nutrition: Calories 48 Fat 1g Carbs 2.5g Protein 9g

3. Fried Cod & Spring Onion

Basic Recipe

Preparation Time: 5 minutes

Cooking Time: 20 minutes

Servings: 4

Ingredients:

- 7-ounce cod fillet, washed and dried
- Spring onion, white and green parts, chopped
- A dash of sesame oil
- 5 tablespoons light soy sauce
- 1 teaspoon dark soy sauce
- 3 tablespoons olive oil
- 5 slices of ginger
- 1 cup of water
- Salt and pepper to taste

Directions:

1. Season the cod fillet with a dash of sesame oil, salt, and pepper. Preheat your air fryer to 356-degreeFahrenheit. Cook the cod fillet in air fryer for 12-minutes

2. For the seasoning sauce, boil water in a pan on the stovetop, along with both light and dark soy sauce and stir.

3. In another small saucepan, heat the oil and add the ginger and white part of the spring onion. Fry until the ginger browns, then remove the ginger and onions.

4. Top the cod fillet with shredded green onion. Pour the oil over the fillet and add the seasoning sauce on top.

Nutrition: Calories 233 Fat 16g Carbs 15.5g Protein 6.7g

4. Medium-Rare Beef Steak

Basic Recipe

Preparation Time: 5 minutes

Cooking Time: 6 minutes

Servings: 4

Ingredients:

- 1-3cm thick beef steak

- 1 tablespoon olive oil

- Salt and pepper to taste

Directions:

1. Preheat your air fryer to 350-degreeFahrenheit.

2. Coat the steak with olive oil on both sides and season both sides with salt and pepper.

3. Place the steak into the baking tray of air fryer and cook for 3-minutes per side.

Nutrition: Calories 445 Fat 21g, Carbs 0g, Protein 59.6g

5. Spicy Duck Legs

Basic Recipe

Preparation Time: 5 minutes

Cooking Time: 30 minutes

Servings: 2

Ingredients:

- 2 duck legs, bone-in, and skin on
- Salt and pepper to taste
- 1 teaspoon five spice powder
- 1 tablespoon herbs that you like such as thyme, parsley, etc., chopped

Directions:

1. Rub the spices over duck legs.
2. Place duck legs in the air fryer and cook for 25-minutes at 325-degreeFahrenheit.
3. Then air fries them at 400-degreeFahrenheit for 5-minutes

Nutrition: Calories 207 Fat 10.6g Carbs 1.9g Protein 25g

6. Stuffed Turkey

Intermediate Recipe

Preparation Time: 5 minutes

Cooking Time: 1hour and 5 minutes

Servings: 4

Ingredients:

- 1 whole turkey, bone-in, with skin
- 2 celery stalks, chopped
- 1 lemon, sliced
- Fresh oregano leaves, chopped
- 1 cup fresh parsley, minced
- 1 teaspoon sage leaves, dry
- 2 cups turkey broth
- 4 cloves garlic, minced
- 1 onion, chopped
- 2 eggs
- 1 ½ lbs. sage sausage
- 4 tablespoons butter

Directions:

1. Preheat your air fryer to 390-degreeFahrenheit. In a pan over medium-heat melt 2 ½ tablespoons of butter. Add the sausage (remove sausage meat from skin) and mash.

2. Cook sausage meat in the pan for 8-minutes and stir. Add in celery, onions, garlic, and sage and cook for an additional 10-minutes, stir to combine.

3. Remove sausage mixture from heat and add the broth. In a bowl, whisk eggs and two tablespoons of parsley.

4. Pour egg mixture into sausage mix and stir. This will be the stuffing for your turkey. Fill the turkey with the stuffing mix. In a separate bowl, combine the remaining butter with parsley, oregano, salt, and pepper and rub this mix onto turkey skin.

5. Place the turkey inside the air fryer and cook for 45-minutes Garnish with lemon slices.

Nutrition: Calories 1046 Fat 69.7g Carbs 12.7g Protein 91.5g

7. Indian Lemon Chili Prawns

Basic Recipe

Preparation Time: 8 minutes

Cooking Time: 15 minutes

Servings: 3

Ingredients:

- 250g of prawns
- Pinch of salt
- ½ tablespoon of ginger garlic paste
- 5ml of lemon juice
- 5g of chili garlic paste
- 50g of hung curd
- A dash of soya sauce
- 10ml of cooking oil

Directions:

1. Remove the veins from the prawns. Wash and dry them. Place to the side for later.

2. In a bowl mix together the salt, ginger garlic paste, lemon juice, chili garlic paste, hung curd, and the soya sauce. Marinate the prawns in the sauce. Leave for one hour.

3. Preheat the Air Fryer to 400 degrees Fahrenheit. Coat the base of the Air Fryer with cooking oil.

4. Put the prawns into the basket and coat lightly with the oil. Cook the prawns for 6 minutes Turnover and cook for another 6 minutes

Nutrition: Calories 148 Fat 4.7g Carbs 2.4g Protein 22.7g

8. Chinese Style White Fish with Sauce

Basic Recipe

Preparation Time: 5 minutes

Cooking Time: 10 minutes

Servings: 2

Ingredients:

- 2 pieces of sway fish fillet
- 1 tablespoon of rice wine
- 2 tablespoons of olive oil
- 2 tablespoons of ginger
- ¼ cup of dark soy sauce
- 2 tablespoons of Shaoxing wine
- ½ teaspoon of salt
- 1 tablespoon of sugar
- 2 green onions
- 1 tablespoon of corn-starch
- 60ml of water

Directions:

1. Firstly, I would recommend lining the bottom of your air fryer basket with lightly greased aluminum foil, you will thank me later when there is less to clean!

2. Make sure that your Swai Fish fillet is defrosted and dry. Cover both sides of the fish with the rice wine and place inside the air fryer basket. For 8-10 minutes cook the fish at 380 degrees Fahrenheit. Make sure to check the fish is cooked through when removing. You can check this by making sure the temperature of the fish is exceeding 145 degrees Fahrenheit.

3. Whilst the fish is cooking, you can create the sauce. For this, you can use a wok. Cut up half of the green onions and add to the wok along with the ginger (This will need to be grated), Sauté these for about 1 minute, you can then add in the soy sauce, Shaoxing wine, salt, and sugar. Bring these to boil.

4. Next, you need a small bowl, mix both the corn starch with the water and pour this into the mixture in your wok stirring until the sauce thickens.

5. When the fish is cooked, you can place the fish onto the serving plate and pour the sauce you've made over the fish. You can use the other half of the green onion to garnish the fish.

Nutrition: Calories 319 Fat 14g Carbs 40g Protein 1g

9. Mexican Shrimp Tacos

Intermediate Recipe

Preparation Time: 20 minutes

Cooking Time: 10 minutes

Servings: 4

Ingredients:

- 1 tablespoon of vegetable oil
- 300g of (raw) shrimps
- 1 ½ teaspoon of light brown sugar
- 1 teaspoon of chipotle chili powder
- ½ teaspoon of smoked paprika
- ½ teaspoon of garlic powder
- ¼ teaspoon of salt
- 130g of fresh avocado
- 130g of purple cabbage
- 60g of green salsa
- 60g of sour cream
- 60g of red onion
- Lime wedges (to serve with)
- 12 street sized flour tortillas

Directions:

1. Firstly, you want to defrost the shrimp according to the package directions. Make sure they are peeled, deveined and without their tails.

2. To prepare the vegetables you are using, you should slice the avocado, chop the cabbage and finely chop the red onion.

3. Preheat the Air Fryer to 400 degrees Fahrenheit, making sure to lightly coat the basket with the vegetable oil.

4. In a bowl, stir together the brown sugar, chipotle chili powder, smoked paprika, garlic powder and the salt.

5. Place the shrimp into a zippered plastic bag and pour in the seasoning mixture you have just prepared. Shake well to ensure the shrimp is evenly covered.

6. Next, put the now seasoned shrimp into the Air Fryer and cook at 400 degrees Fahrenheit for 3 to 4 minutes Turn each shrimp over and cook for an additional 3-4 minutes

7. When fully cooked, mix the shrimps with the green salsa and sour cream. Place into the flour tortillas and add the avocado, cabbage, red onion and a squeeze of lime.

Nutrition: Calories 470 Fat 31.6g Carbs 38g Protein 11g

10. Thai Fish Cakes

Intermediate Recipe

Preparation Time: 20 minutes

Cooking Time: 15 minutes

Servings: 4

Ingredients:

- 130g of mash potatoes
- 260g of white fish
- 1 small onion
- 1 teaspoon of butter
- 1 teaspoon of milk – will need extra for poaching
- 1 lime
- 3 teaspoons of chili
- 1 teaspoon of Worcester sauce
- 1 teaspoon of coriander
- 1 teaspoon of mixed spice
- 1 teaspoon of mixed herbs
- Breadcrumbs
- Salt & pepper

Directions:

1. Place the white fish into a large pan and cover with the milk.

2. Once covered with milk, dry out the fish of the milk and put into a large mixing bowl. Add the chili, mixed herbs, mixed spice, coriander, Worcester sauce, lime, salt and pepper and the onion, along with the mash potatoes and mix well. Once mixed, mash to ensure there are no lumps

3. Add the butter and milk and mix well together.

4. Form into small fishcakes using the breadcrumbs and place into the fridge for 3 hours.

5. Once the 3 hours is up, put into the air fryer and cook at 400 degrees Fahrenheit for 15 minutes, making sure to turn them over halfway through.

Nutrition: Calories 317 Fat 25.1g Carbs 11.4g Protein 12.2g

11. Wondrous Creole Fried Shrimp with Sriracha Sauce

Basic Recipe

Preparation Time: 10 minutes

Cooking Time: 10 minutes

Servings: 4

Ingredients:

- 1 pound of peeled and deveined shrimp
- ½ cup of cornmeal
- ½ cup of breadcrumbs
- 1 beaten egg
- 1 tablespoon of hot sauce
- 1 tablespoon of mustard
- 2 tablespoons of creole seasoning
- 1 teaspoon of onion powder
- 1 teaspoon of garlic powder
- 1 teaspoon of black pepper
- 1 teaspoon of salt

- Siracha sauce ingredients

- 1 cup of mayonnaise

- 3 tablespoons of sriracha sauce

- 1 tablespoon of soy sauce

- 1 teaspoon of black pepper

Directions:

1. Turn on your air fryer to 360 degrees Fahrenheit.

2. Using a bowl, add the eggs, hot sauce, mustard, 1 tablespoon of creole seasoning, onion powder, garlic powder, black pepper, salt, the shrimp and toss until it is properly covered.

3. Using another bowl, add the breadcrumbs, flour, 1 tablespoon of creole seasoning, and the shrimp and cover it properly.

4. Grease your air fryer basket with a nonstick cooking spray and add the shrimp.

5. Cook it for 5 minutes or until it has a golden-brown color, while being careful not to overcook.

6. Thereafter, carefully remove it from your air fryer and allow it to cool.

7. Pick a separate bowl, add and mix all the sauce ingredients properly. Serve!

Nutrition: Calories 200 Fat 12g Protein 15gCarbs 7g

12. **Buttered Scallops**

Basic Recipe

Preparation Time: 10 minutes

Cooking Time: 5 minutes

Servings: 8

Ingredients:

- 4 tablespoons butter, melted
- 3-pounds Sea scallops
- 2 tablespoons fresh thyme, minced
- Salt and freshly ground black pepper, to taste

Directions:

1. Add butter, sea scallops, thyme, salt and pepper in a bowl. Toss to coat well.
2. Preheat the air fryer to 385 degrees F and grease the air fryer basket.
3. Place scallops in the basket and cook for 5 minutes
4. Take out and serve hot.
5. Tip: Pour melted butter on the scallops to enhance their taste.

Nutrition: Calories 203 Fat 7.1g Carbs 4.5g Protein 28.7g

13. Ham Wrapped Prawns

Basic Recipe

Preparation Time: 15 minutes

Cooking Time: 15 minutes

Servings: 4

Ingredients:

- 2 garlic cloves, minced
- 1 tablespoon paprika
- 8 king prawns, peeled, deveined and chopped
- 4 ham slices, halved
- 2 tablespoons olive oil
- Salt and freshly ground black pepper, to taste

Directions:

1. Preheat the air fryer to 430 degrees F and wrap each prawn with a ham slice.
2. Arrange in the air fryer basket and cook for about 4 minutes
3. Dish out and meanwhile place bell pepper in the air fryer basket.
4. Cook for about 10 minutes and transfer in a bowl.
5. Cover the bowl with a foil and set aside for 15 minutes

6. Now, place bell pepper, garlic, paprika and oil in a blender.

7. Blend till a puree is formed and serve with ham wrapped prawns.

Nutrition: Calories 553 Fat 33.6g Carbs 2.6g Protein 5g

14. Nacho Chips Crusted Prawns

Basic Recipe

Preparation Time: 10 minutes

Cooking Time: 10 minutes

Servings: 8

Ingredients:

- 2 large eggs

- 36 prawns, peeled and deveined

- 1½-pounds Nacho flavored chips, crushed finely

Directions:

1. Add nacho chips in a bowl and crush well.

2. Add eggs in another bowl and beat well.

3. Preheat the air fryer to 350 degrees F.

4. Dip each prawn in the egg mixture and then in the crushed nachos.

5. Place them in the air fryer and cook for about 8 minutes

6. Take out and serve hot.

Tip: More crushed nachos will make prawns crispier.

Nutrition: Calories 1090 Fat 55.2g Carbs 101.9g Protein 49.2g

15. Spicy Shrimp

Basic Recipe

Preparation Time: 5 minutes

Cooking Time: 5 minutes

Servings: 8

Ingredients:

- 2 teaspoons old bay seasoning
- 1 teaspoon cayenne pepper
- 1 teaspoon smoked paprika
- 4 tablespoons olive oil
- 2-pounds tiger shrimp
- Salt, to taste

Directions:

1. Add all the ingredients in a large bowl. Mix well. Preheat the air fryer to 390 degrees F and grease the air fryer basket.
2. Place shrimps in the air fryer basket and cook for about 5 minutes. Take out and serve hot.

Tip: Top with chili sauce to enhance its taste.

Nutrition: Calories 174 Fat 8.3g Carbs 0.3g Protein 23.8g

16. Lemon Tuna

Basic Recipe

Preparation Time: 10 minutes

Cooking Time: 12 minutes

Servings: 4

Ingredients:

- 1 tablespoon fresh lime juice
- 1 egg
- 3 tablespoons canola oil
- 2 tablespoons hot sauce
- 2 teaspoons Dijon mustard
- 2 tablespoons fresh parsley, chopped
- ½ pound water packed plain tuna
- ½ cup breadcrumbs
- Salt and freshly ground black pepper, to taste

Directions:

1. Add tuna fish, parsley, mustard, crumbs, citrus juice and hot sauce in a bowl. Mix well.
2. Now, add oil, salt and eggs in the bowl and make patties from the mixture.
3. Refrigerate and preheat the air fryer to 360 degrees F.

4. Place the patties in the air fryer basket and cook for 12 minutes

5. Take out and serve hot.

Nutrition: Calories 315 Fat 18.7g Carbs 25g Protein 10.7g

17. Lemony & Spicy Coconut Crusted Prawns

Basic Recipe

Preparation Time: 20 minutes

Cooking Time: 7 minutes

Servings: 4

Ingredients:

- ½ cup unsweetened coconut, shredded
- ¼ teaspoon lemon zest
- ¼ teaspoon cayenne pepper
- Vegetable oil, as required
- ¼ teaspoon red pepper flakes, crushed
- ½ cup flour
- ½ cup breadcrumbs
- 1-pound prawns, peeled and de-veined
- 2 egg whites
- Salt and black pepper, to taste

Directions:

1. Take a shallow dish and mix salt, flour and pepper in it.
2. Crack eggs in another shallow dish. Beat well.

3. In the third shallow dish, add coconut, breadcrumbs, lime zest, salt and cayenne pepper. Mix well.

4. Now, preheat the air fryer to 395 degrees F.

5. Dip shrimp into flour mixture, then in the egg mixture and roll them evenly into the breadcrumb mixture.

6. Place them in the air fryer basket and Drizzle with vegetable oil over them.

7. Cook for about 7 minutes and take out.

8. Serve and enjoy!

Nutrition: Calories 773 Fat 60.7g Carbs 25.5g Protein 31.5g

18. Tuna Stuffed Potatoes

Basic Recipe

Preparation Time: 15 minutes

Cooking Time: 30 minutes

Servings: 4

Ingredients:

- 1½-pounds tuna, Dry out
- 2 tablespoons plain Greek yogurt
- ½ tablespoon olive oil
- 4 starchy potatoes, soaked for 30 minutes
- 1 tablespoon capers
- 1 teaspoon red chili powder
- 1 scallion, chopped and divided
- Salt and freshly ground black pepper, to taste

Directions:

1. Preheat the air fryer to 355 degrees F.
2. Place the potatoes in the air fryer basket and cook for about 30 minutes
3. Take out and place on a flat surface.
4. Meanwhile, add yogurt, tuna, red chili powder, scallion, salt and pepper in a bowl. Mix well.

5. Cut each potato from top side lengthwise and press the open side of potato halves slightly.

6. Stuff potato with tuna mixture and sprinkle with capers.

7. Dish out and serve.

Nutrition: Calories 1387 Fat 54g Carbs 35.7g Protein 180.7g

19. Cajun Spiced Salmon

Basic Recipe

Preparation Time: 10 minutes

Cooking Time: 10 minutes

Servings: 8

Ingredients:

- 4 tablespoons Cajun seasoning
- 4 salmon steaks

Directions:

1. Add Cajun seasoning in a bowl and rub salmon evenly with it.
2. Preheat the air fryer to 385 degrees F.
3. Arrange air fryer grill pan and place salmon steaks on it.
4. Cook for about 8 minutes and flip once in the middle way.
5. Take out and serve hot.

Nutrition: Calories 118 Fat 5.5g Carbs 0g Protein 17.3g

20. Tangy Salmon

Basic Recipe

Preparation Time: 10 minutes

Cooking Time: 10 minutes

Servings: 8

Ingredients:

- 4 tablespoons Cajun seasoning
- 8 salmon fillets
- 4 tablespoons fresh lemon juice

Directions:

1. Season salmon fillets with Cajun seasoning and set aside for 15 minutes
2. Preheat the air fryer to 360 degrees F and arrange grill pan in it.
3. Place salmon fillets on the grill pan and cook for about 7 minutes
4. Drizzle with lemon juice and serve.

Nutrition: Calories 237 Fat 11.1g Carbs 21gProtein 34.7g

21. **Crispy Crust Ranch Fish Fillets**

Preparation Time: 10 minutes

Cooking Time: 12 minutes

Serving: 2

Ingredients:

- 2 fish fillets
- 1/2 packet ranch dressing mix
- 1/4 cup breadcrumbs
- 1 egg, lightly beaten
- 1 1/4 tbsp olive oil

Directions:

1. In a shallow dish mix together ranch dressing mix and breadcrumbs.
2. Add oil and mix until the mixture becomes crumbly.
3. Place the dehydrating tray in a multi-level air fryer basket and place basket in the instant pot.
4. Dip fish fillet in egg then coats with breadcrumb and place on dehydrating tray.

5. Seal pot with air fryer lid and select air fry mode then set the temperature to 350 F and timer for 12 minutes. Turn fish fillets halfway through.

6. Serve and enjoy.

Nutrition: Calories 373 Fat 22.9 g Carbohydrates 25.7 g Sugar 1.2 g Protein 18 g Cholesterol 113 mg

22. **Steam Shrimp**

Preparation Time: 10 minutes

Cooking Time: 6 minutes

Serving: 4

Ingredients:

- 2 lbs. shrimp, cleaned
- 1 1/2 tsp old bay seasoning
- 1 tsp Cajun seasoning
- Pepper
- Salt

Directions:

1. Add all ingredients into the inner pot of air fryer and stir well.
2. Seal the pot with pressure cooking lid and select steam mode and cook for 6 minutes.
3. Once done, release pressure using a quick release. Remove lid.
4. Stir well and serve.

Nutrition: Calories 270 Fat 3.8 g Carbohydrates 3.5 g Sugar 0 g Protein 51.7 g Cholesterol 478 mg

23. <u>Delicious Shrimp Paella</u>

Preparation Time: 10 minutes

Cooking Time: 5 minutes

Serving: 4

Ingredients:

- 1 lb. jumbo shrimp, frozen
- 1/2 cup white wine
- 1 cup fish broth
- 1 red pepper, chopped
- 4 garlic cloves, chopped
- 1 onion, chopped
- 1/4 butter
- 1 cup of rice
- 1/4 cup cilantro, chopped
- 1/4 tsp red pepper flakes
- 1 tsp turmeric
- 1 tsp paprika
- 1/4 tsp pepper
- 1/2 tsp salt

Directions:

1. Add butter into the inner pot of air fryer and set pot on sauté mode.
2. Add garlic and onion and cook for a minute.
3. Add remaining ingredients and stir well.
4. Seal the pot with pressure cooking lid and cook on high for 5 minutes.
5. Once done, release pressure using a quick release. Remove lid.
6. Serve and enjoy.

Nutrition: Calories 310 Fat 1.3 g Carbohydrates 44.4 g Sugar 5.1 g Protein 24.6 g Cholesterol 235 mg

24. Crispy Coconut Shrimp

Preparation Time: 10 minutes

Cooking Time: 10 minutes

Serving: 2

Ingredients:

- 12 large shrimp
- 1 cup coconut, dried
- 1 cup flour
- 1 cup breadcrumbs
- 1 cup egg white
- 1 tbsp cornstarch

Directions:

1. In a shallow dish, mix together coconut and breadcrumbs and set aside.
2. In another dish, mix together flour and cornstarch and set aside.
3. Add egg white in a small bowl.
4. Line instant pot multi-level air fryer basket with aluminum foil.
5. Dip shrimp in egg white then roll in flour and coat with breadcrumb.

6. Place coated shrimp into the air fryer basket and place basket into the instant pot.

7. Seal pot with air fryer lid and select air fry mode then set the temperature to 350 F and timer for 10 minutes. Turn shrimp halfway through.

8. Serve and enjoy.

Nutrition: Calories 700 Fat 17.6 g Carbohydrates 97.7 g Sugar 6.9 g Protein 35.8 g Cholesterol 69 mg

25. Cheesy Shrimp Grits

Preparation time: 10 minutes

Cooking time: 7 minutes

Servings: 6

Ingredients:

- 1 lb. shrimp, thawed
- 1/2 cup cheddar cheese, shredded
- 1/2 cup quick grits
- 1 tbsp butter
- 1 1/2 cups chicken broth
- 1/4 tsp red pepper flakes
- 1/2 tsp paprika
- 2 tbsp cilantro, chopped
- 1 tbsp coconut oil
- 1/2 tsp kosher salt

Directions:

1. Add oil into the instant pot and set the pot on sauté mode.
2. Add shrimp and cook until shrimp is no longer pink. Season with red pepper flakes and salt.
3. Remove shrimp from the pot and set aside.

4. Add remaining ingredients into the pot and stir well.

5. Seal pot with lid and cook on manual high pressure for 7 minutes.

6. Once done then allow to release pressure naturally then open the lid.

7. Stir in cheese and top with shrimp.

Nutrition: Calories 221 Fat 9.1 g Carbohydrates 12 g Sugar 0.3 g Protein 21.9 g Cholesterol 174 mg

26. Curried Salmon Patties

Preparation Time: 10 minutes

Cooking Time: 8 minutes

Serving: 6

Ingredients:

- 14 oz can salmon, drained & remove bones
- 1/2 lime zest
- 1 tbsp brown sugar
- 2 eggs, lightly beaten
- 2 tbsp red curry paste
- 1/2 cup breadcrumbs
- 1/4 tsp salt

Directions:

1. Add all ingredients into the bowl and mix until well combined.
2. Place the dehydrating tray in a multi-level air fryer basket and place basket in the instant pot.
3. Make patties from mixture and place on dehydrating tray.

4. Seal pot with air fryer lid and select air fry mode then set the temperature to 400 F and timer for 8 minutes. Turn patties halfway through.
5. Serve and enjoy.

Nutrition: Calories 174 Fat 7.4 g Carbohydrates 9.1 g Sugar 2.2 g Protein 16.1 g Cholesterol 91 mg

27. Fish Finger Sandwich in Instant Pot Air Fryer

Preparation: 5 minutes

Cooking: 15 minutes

Servings: 4

Ingredients:

- 13 ounces (4 Nos.) cod fillet, skin removed
- 2 tablespoons flour
- 1½ ounce breadcrumbs
- 12 capers
- 10 ounces of frozen peas
- 1 tablespoon Greek yogurt
- 1 tablespoon lemon juice
- 8 small slices of bread
- ¼ teaspoon salt
- ½ teaspoon ground black pepper
- Cooking oil spray

Directions:

1. Wash the fillets and pat dry.
2. Close the crisp cover of the Instant Pot Air Fryer and set the temperature to 390°F.

3. Set the timer 5 minutes and press start for preheating in AIR FRY mode.

4. Rub salt and pepper on all sides of the fillets.

5. Place the flour in a medium shallow bowl.

6. Similarly, place the breadcrumbs in a shallow bowl.

7. Now dredge the cod fillets in the flour and then dredge in the breadcrumbs.

8. Spray some cooking in the instant fryer basket and place the cod fillets in it.

9. Place the basket in the inner pot of the Instant Pot.

10. Close the crisp cover and keep the temperature at 390°F in AIR FRY mode.

11. Set the timer to 15 minutes and press START for air frying.

12. When the cooking is under process, boil the peas for 5 minutes until it becomes tender.

13. Once it becomes tender, drain it and put it in a blender.

14. Add capers, Greek yogurt, and lemon juice.

15. Blitz the ingredients until it blends thoroughly.

16. After finish cooking, remove the fillets from the Instant Pot Air Fryer and layer it for making the sandwich.

17. Over the bread slice, layer fish fillet and spread the pea puree.

18. Serve warm.

Nutrition: Calories: 458, Total Fat: 18.8g, Saturated fat: 3.2g, Trans fat: 0g, Cholesterol: 0mg, Sodium: 1516mg, Total carbs: 44g, Dietary fiber: 10g, Sugars: 7g, Protein: 29g

28. Shrimp Parmesan Bake

Preparation time: 10 minutes

Cooking time: 8 minutes

Servings: 4

Ingredients:

- 1 1/2 lb. Large raw shrimp, peeled and deveined
- 1/4 cup melted butter
- 1 teaspoon coarse salt
- 1/4 teaspoon black pepper
- 1 teaspoon garlic powder
- 1/2 teaspoon crushed red pepper
- 1/4 cup parmesan cheese, grated

Directions:

1. Toss the shrimp with oil and all other ingredients in a bowl.
2. Spread the seasoned shrimp in the baking tray.
3. Press "power button" of air fry oven and turn the dial to select the "bake" mode.
4. Press the time button and again turn the dial to set the cooking time to 8 minutes.

5. Now push the temp button and rotate the dial to set the temperature at 400 degrees f.

6. Once preheated, place the lobster's baking tray in the oven and close its lid.

7. Switch the air fryer oven to broil mode and cook for 1 minute.

8. Serve warm.

Nutrition: Calories 231 Total fat 14.9g Saturated fat 7.6g Cholesterol 249mg Sodium 1058mg Total carbohydrate 2.3g Dietary fiber 0.2g Total sugars 0.2g Protein 23.3g

29. <u>Honey Mustard Salmon</u>

Preparation Time: 10 minutes

Cooking Time: 9 minutes

Serving: 2

Ingredients:

- 2 salmon fillets
- 2 tbsp Dijon mustard
- 2 tbsp honey
- 1/4 cup mayonnaise
- Pepper
- Salt

Directions:

1. In a small bowl, mix together mustard, honey, mayonnaise, pepper, and salt and brush over salmon.
2. Place the dehydrating tray in a multi-level air fryer basket and place basket in the instant pot.
3. Place salmon fillets on dehydrating tray.
4. Seal pot with air fryer lid and select air fry mode then set the temperature to 350 F and timer for 9 minutes.
5. Serve and enjoy.

Nutrition: Calories 424 Fat 21.4 g Carbohydrates 25.2 g Sugar 19.3 g Protein 35.5 g Cholesterol 86 mg

30. Bacon-Wrapped Shrimp

Preparation time:10 minutes

Cooking Time: 10 minutes

Serving: 6

Ingredients:

- 1-pound shrimp
- 1 package bacon
- 1/2 teaspoon cayenne pepper
- 1/2 teaspoon ground cumin
- 1/2 teaspoon onion powder
- 1/2 teaspoon lemon zest
- 1 teaspoon garlic powder
- 1 tablespoon Worcestershire sauce
- 1 tablespoon lemon juice

Directions:

1. Whisk Worcestershire sauce with cayenne pepper, onion powder, cumin, lemon zest, and garlic powder in a large bowl.

2. Toss in shrimp and mix well to coat then cover them to refrigerate for 1 hour.

3. Cut the bacon in half and wrap each half around each shrimp.

4. Place the wrapped shrimp in the Air Fryer Basket and set it in the Instant Pot Duo.

5. Put on the Air Fryer lid and seal it.

6. Hit the "Air fry Button" and select 10 minutes of cooking time, then press "Start."

7. Once the Instant Pot Duo beeps, remove its lid.

8. Serve.

Nutrition: Calories 114 Total Fat 2.7g Saturated Fat 0.9g Cholesterol 163mg Sodium 286mg Total Carbohydrate 2.4g Dietary Fiber 0.1g Total Sugars 0.8g Protein 18.6g

31. Horseradish Crusted Salmon

Preparation time:10 minutes

Cooking Time: 5 minutes

Serving: 2

Ingredients:

- 2 pieces of salmon fillet
- 1 teaspoon salt
- 1 teaspoon black pepper
- 1 tablespoon horseradish
- 2 tablespoons olive oil
- 1/4 cup bread crumbs

Directions:

1. Whisk bread crumbs with salt, olive oil, horseradish and black pepper in a bowl.
2. Coat the salmon with this crumbly mixture liberally.
3. Place the breaded salmon in the Air Fryer Basket and set it inside the Instant Pot Duo.
4. Put on the Air Fryer lid and seal it.
5. Hit the "Air fry Button" and select 5 minutes of cooking time, then press "Start."

6. Once the Instant Pot Duo beeps, remove its lid.

7. Serve.

Nutrition: Calories 415 Total Fat 25.8g Saturated Fat 3.8g Cholesterol 78mg Sodium 1364mg Total Carbohydrate 11.3g Dietary Fiber 1.1g Total Sugars 1.5g Protein 36.5g

32. <u>Air Fryer Roast Beef</u>

Preparation: 5 minutes

Cooking time: 15 minutes

Servings: 6

Ingredients:

- 2½ pound beef
- 1 tablespoon Montreal steak seasoning
- 1 tablespoon olive oil

Directions:

1. Tie up the beef to make it compact enough to cook.
2. Rub some olive oil all over the beef roast
3. Sprinkle the seasoning over the meat.
4. Put the air fryer basket in the inner pot of the instant pot air fryer.
5. Place the separator in the air fryer basket and keep the beef on the separator.
6. Close the crisp cover.
7. Select the smart option roast under air fryer and set the timer to 15 minutes.

8. Press the start button and let the meat cook well.

9. Open the crisp cover and flip it halfway through for even cooking.

10. After flipping close the crisp cover again to resume cooking for the remaining period.

11. Once done, allow it to rest for 5 minutes before you serve.

Nutrition: Calories 276, total fat: 13g, saturated fat: 3.4g, trans fat: 0.6g, cholesterol: 140mg, sodium: 266mg, total carbs: 1g, dietary fiber: 0g, sugars: 0g, protein: 39g.

33. Smoked Lamb Chops

Preparation time: 25 minutes

Cooking time: 10 minutes

Servings: 4

Ingredients:

- 4 lamb chops
- 4 garlic cloves; minced
- 2 tbsp. Olive oil
- ¼ tsp. Smoked paprika
- ½ tsp. Chili powder
- A pinch of salt and black pepper

Directions:

1. Take a bowl and mix the lamb with the rest of the ingredients and toss well
2. Transfer the chops to your air fryer's basket and cook at 390°f for 10 minutes on each side. Serve with a side salad

Nutrition: Calories: 274; Fat: 12g; Fiber: 4g; Carbs: 6g; Protein: 17g

34. **Spicy Beef**

Preparation time: 25 minutes

Cooking time: 10 minutes

Servings: 4

Ingredients:

- 4 beef steaks
- 1 tbsp. Hot paprika
- 1 tbsp. Butter; melted
- Salt and black pepper to taste.

Directions:

1. Take a bowl and mix the beef with the rest of the ingredients, rub well, transfer the steaks to your air fryer's basket and cook at 390°f for 10 minutes on each side

2. Divide the steaks between plates and serve with a side salad.

Nutrition: Calories: 280; Fat: 12g; Fiber: 4g; Carbs: 6g; Protein: 17g

35. <u>Adobo Beef</u>

Preparation time: 35 minutes

Cooking time: 10 minutes

Servings: 4

Ingredients:

- 1 lb. Beef roast, trimmed
- 1 tbsp. Olive oil
- ¼ tsp. Garlic powder
- ½ tsp. Turmeric powder
- ½ tsp. Oregano; dried
- A pinch of salt and black pepper

Directions:

1. Take a bowl and mix the roast with the rest of the ingredients and rub well.
2. Put the roast in the air fryer's basket and cook at 390°f for 30 minutes.
3. Slice the roast, divide it between plates and serve with a side salad.

Nutrition: Calories: 294; Fat: 12g; Fiber: 3g; Carbs: 6g; Protein: 19g

36. __Pork Chop Salad__

Preparation time: 23 minutes

Cooking time: 10 minutes

Servings: 2

Ingredients:

- 2 (4-oz. pork chops; chopped into 1-inch cubes
- ½ cup shredded Monterey jack cheese
- 1 medium avocado; peeled, pitted and diced
- ¼ cup full-fat ranch dressing
- 4 cups chopped romaine
- 1 medium roma tomato; diced
- 1 tbsp. Chopped cilantro
- 1 tbsp. Coconut oil
- ½ tsp. Garlic powder.
- ¼ tsp. Onion powder.
- 2 tsp. Chili powder
- 1 tsp. Paprika

Directions:

1. Take a large bowl, drizzle coconut oil over pork.
2. Sprinkle with chili powder, paprika, garlic powder and onion powder.

3. Place pork into the air fryer basket.

4. Adjust the temperature to 400 degrees f and set the timer for 8 minutes.

5. Pork will be golden and crispy when fully cooked

6. Take a large bowl, place romaine, tomato and crispy pork.

7. Top with shredded cheese and avocado.

8. Pour ranch dressing around bowl and toss the salad to evenly coat.

9. Top with cilantro.

10. Serve immediately.

Nutrition: Calories: 526; Protein: 34.4g; Fiber: 8.6g; Fat: 37.0g; Carbs: 13.8g

37. **Fajita Flank Steak Rolls**

Preparation time: 35 minutes

Cooking time: 10 minutes

Servings: 6

Ingredients:

- 2 lb. Flank steak
- 4 (1-oz. slices pepper jack cheese
- 1 medium red bell pepper; seeded and sliced into strips
- ¼ cup diced yellow onion
- 1 medium green bell pepper; seeded and sliced into strips
- 2 tbsp. Unsalted butter.
- 1 tsp. Cumin
- ½ tsp. Garlic powder.
- 2 tsp. Chili powder

Directions:

1. In a medium skillet over medium heat, melt butter and begin sautéing onion, red bell pepper and green bell pepper. Sprinkle with chili powder, cumin and garlic powder. Sauté until peppers are tender, about 5–7 minutes.

2. Lay flank steak flat on a work surface. Spread onion and pepper mixture over entire steak rectangle. Lay slices of cheese on top of onions and peppers, barely overlapping

3. With the shortest end toward you, begin rolling the steak, tucking the cheese down into the roll as necessary.

4. Secure the roll with twelve toothpicks, six on each side of the steak roll. Place steak roll into the air fryer basket

5. Adjust the temperature to 400 degrees f and set the timer for 15 minutes. Rotate the roll halfway through the cooking time. Add an additional 1–4 minutes depending on your preferred internal temperature (135 degrees f for medium

6. When timer beeps, allow roll to rest 15 minutes, then slice into six even pieces.

7. Serve warm.

Nutrition: Calories: 439; Protein: 38.0g; Fiber: 1.2g; Fat: 26.6g; Carbs: 3.7g

38. Moroccan Lamb

Preparation time: 35 minutes

Cooking time: 10 minutes

Servings: 4

Ingredients:

- 8 lamb cutlets
- ½ cup mint leaves
- 6 garlic cloves
- 3 tbsp. Lemon juice
- 1 tbsp. Coriander seeds
- 4 tbsp. Olive oil
- 1 tbsp. Cumin, ground
- Zest of 2 lemons, grated
- A pinch of salt and black pepper

Directions:

1. In a blender, combine all the ingredients except the lamb and pulse well.
2. Rub the lamb cutlets with this mix, place them in your air fryer's basket and cook at 380°f for 15 minutes on each side.

3. Serve with a side salad

Nutrition: Calories: 284; Fat: 13g; Fiber: 3g; Carbs: 5g; Protein: 15g

39. Cuban Pork

Preparation Time: 10 minutes

Cooking Time: 8 hours 10 minutes

Serving: 6

Ingredients:

- 3 lbs. pork shoulder roast
- 1 tsp oregano, dried
- 1 tsp cumin
- 1/2 cup fresh lime juice
- 1/2 cup orange juice
- 1 bay leaf
- 1 onion, sliced
- 1 1/2 garlic cloves, crushed
- 1/4 tsp red chili flakes
- 2 tbsp olive oil
- 1/8 tsp pepper
- 1 1/2 tsp salt

Directions:

1. In a bowl, mix together garlic, pepper, chili flakes, lime juice, orange juice, oil, oregano, cumin, and salt,

2. Place pork into the inner pot of air fryer . Pour bowl mixture over pork.

3. Add bay leaf. Seal the pot with pressure cooking lid and select slow cook mode and cook on low for 8 hours.

4. Remove meat from pot and shred using a fork.

5. Clean the pot. Add shredded meat into the air fryer basket and place basket into the pot.

6. Seal the pot with air fryer lid and select broil mode and cook for 10 minutes.

7. Serve and enjoy.

Nutrition: Calories 644 Fat 51 g Carbohydrates 5 g Sugar 2.6 g Protein 38.7 g Cholesterol 161 mg

40. Pork Tenderloin

Preparation Time: 10 minutes

Cooking Time: 6 hours

Serving: 8

Ingredients:

- 2 lbs. pork tenderloin
- 1/2 cup balsamic vinegar
- 1 tbsp garlic cloves, minced
- 1/2 tsp red chili flakes
- 2 tbsp coconut amino
- 1 tbsp Worcestershire sauce
- 1 tbsp olive oil
- 1/2 tsp sea salt

Directions:

1. Add olive oil, garlic, and pork tenderloin into the inner pot of air fryer and set pot on sauté mode.
2. In a bowl, mix together remaining ingredients and pour over pork.
3. Seal the pot with pressure cooking lid and select slow cook mode and cook on low for 6 hours.
4. Serve and enjoy.

Nutrition: Calories 188 Fat 5.7 g Carbohydrates 1.6 g Sugar 0.5 g Protein 29.8 g Cholesterol 83 mg

41. Crispy Mac & Cheese

Preparation Time: 10 minutes

Cooking Time: 9 minutes

Servings: 6

Ingredients:

- 2 1/2 cups macaroni
- 1/4 tsp garlic powder
- 1 sleeve Ritz crackers, crushed
- 1/3 cup parmesan cheese, shredded
- 2 2/3 cups pepper jack cheese, shredded
- 1/2 cup butter, melted
- 1 1/4 cup heavy cream
- 2 cups vegetable broth
- Pepper
- Salt

Directions:

1. Add 1/4 cup butter, broth, garlic powder, cream, pepper, and salt into the instant pot and stir well.

2. Add macaroni and secure pot with pressure cooking lid and cook on high for 4 minutes.

3. Once done, release pressure using quick release. Remove lid.

4. Add 2 cups pepper jack cheese and stir until cheese is melted.

5. Mix together remaining melted butter and crushed crackers sprinkle on top of macaroni.

6. Sprinkle remaining pepper jack cheese and parmesan cheese on top of macaroni.

7. Secure pot with air fryer lid and cook on air fry mode at 400 F for 5 minutes.

8. Serve and enjoy.

Nutrition: Calories 561 Fat 41.1 g Carbohydrates 29.3 g Sugar 1.6 g Protein 19.2 g Cholesterol 124 mg

42. Healthy Ratatouille Pasta

Preparation Time: 10 minutes

Cooking Time: 10 minutes

Servings: 4

Ingredients:

- 1 1/4 cups elbow pasta
- 2 cups vegetable stock
- 14 oz can tomato, chopped
- 1/2 eggplant, chopped
- 1 red bell pepper, diced
- 1 zucchini, chopped
- 1 tsp olive oil
- 1/2 cup parmesan cheese, shredded
- Pepper
- Salt

Directions:

1. Add oil into the instant pot and set the pot on sauté mode.
2. Add eggplant, bell pepper, zucchini, pepper, and salt, and sauté for 5 minutes. Cancel sauté mode.

3. Add pasta, stock, and tomatoes and stir well.

4. Secure pot with pressure cooking lid and cook on high for 2 minutes.

5. Once done, release pressure using quick release. Remove lid.

6. Sprinkle shredded parmesan cheese on top of pasta.

7. Secure pot with air fryer lid and broil for 4 minutes.

8. Serve and enjoy.

Nutrition: Calories 168 Fat 4.2 g Carbohydrates 26.3 g Sugar 8.4 g Protein 8.4 g Cholesterol 8 mg

43. **Healthy & Crispy Broccoli**

Preparation Time: 10 minutes

Cooking Time: 8 minutes

Servings: 2

Ingredients:

- 3 cups broccoli florets
- 1/4 tsp garlic powder
- 2 tbsp olive oil
- 1/8 tsp red chili flakes
- 1/4 tsp pepper
- 1/4 tsp salt

Directions:

1. Add broccoli florets and remaining ingredients into the mixing bowl and toss to combine.
2. Add broccoli florets into the multi-level air fryer basket.
3. Place basket into the pot. Secure pot with air fryer lid and cook on air fry mode at 375 F for 8 minutes.
4. Serve and enjoy.

Nutrition: Calories 168 Fat 14.5 g Carbohydrates 9.5 g Sugar 2.4 g Protein 3.9 g Cholesterol 0 mg

44. Crispy Cauliflower Florets

Preparation Time: 10 minutes

Cooking Time: 10 minutes

Servings: 2

Ingredients:

- 3 cups cauliflower florets
- 1 tbsp almond flour
- 1/4 tsp red chili flakes
- 1/4 tsp garlic powder
- 1 tbsp olive oil
- 1/4 tsp pepper
- Salt

Directions:

1. Add cauliflower florets and remaining ingredients into the bowl and mix well.
2. Add cauliflower florets into the multi-level air fryer basket.
3. Place basket into the pot. Secure pot with air fryer lid and cook on air fry mode at 400 F for 10 minutes.
4. Serve and enjoy.

Nutrition: Calories 179 Fat 14.2 g Carbohydrates 11.4 g Sugar 4.2 g Protein 6.1 g Cholesterol 0 mg

45. <u>Crispy Cauliflower Steaks</u>

Preparation Time: 10 minutes

Cooking Time: 15 minutes

Servings: 4

Ingredients:

- 1 medium cauliflower head, cut into 1-inch-thick slices
- 1 tbsp fresh lime juice
- 1 tsp garlic, minced
- 1/2 tsp paprika
- 1/2 tsp turmeric
- 1 tbsp olive oil
- 1/2 tsp salt

Directions:

1. In a bowl, mix lime juice, garlic, paprika, turmeric, oil, and salt.
2. Add cauliflower slices and coat well and let them sit for 1 hour.
3. Place marinated cauliflower slices into the multi-level air fryer basket.
4. Place basket into the pot. Secure pot with air fryer lid and cook on air fry mode at 375 F for 15 minutes.

5. Serve and enjoy.

Nutrition: Calories 71 Fat 3.7 g Carbohydrates 9.1 g Sugar 3.7 g Protein 3 g Cholesterol 0 mg

46. <u>Roasted Cauliflower</u>

Preparation Time: 10 minutes

Cooking Time: 10 minutes

Servings: 2

Ingredients:

- 3 cups cauliflower florets
- 1 tbsp fresh parsley, chopped
- 1/2 tsp fresh lime juice
- 1/2 tsp dried oregano
- 1 1/2 tbsp olive oil
- 1 tbsp pine nuts
- Pepper
- Salt

Directions:

1. Add cauliflower florets, olive oil, oregano, pepper, and salt into the bowl and toss well.
2. Add cauliflower florets into the multi-level air fryer basket.
3. Place basket into the pot. Secure pot with air fryer lid and cook on air fry mode at 375 F for 10 minutes.

4. Transfer cauliflower florets into the mixing bowl. Add parsley, lime juice, and pine nuts and toss well.

5. Serve and enjoy.

Nutrition: Calories 161 Fat 13.7 g Carbohydrates 9.8 g Sugar 4 g Protein 3.7 g Cholesterol 0 mg

47. Perfect Mexican Cauliflower

Preparation Time: 10 minutes

Cooking Time: 12 minutes

Servings: 4

Ingredients:

- 1 medium cauliflower head, cut into florets
- 1 tsp chili powder
- 1/2 tsp paprika
- 1/2 tsp onion powder
- 1/2 tsp turmeric
- 2 tsp parsley, chopped
- 1 tsp cumin
- 2 tbsp olive oil
- 1 lime juice
- 1 1/2 tsp garlic powder
- Pepper
- Salt

Directions:

1. Add cauliflower florets and remaining ingredients into the mixing bowl and toss well.

2. Add cauliflower florets into the multi-level air fryer basket.

3. Place basket into the pot. Secure pot with air fryer lid and cook on air fry mode at 400 F for 12 minutes.

4. Drizzle with lime juice and serve.

Nutrition: Calories 109 Fat 7.5 g Carbohydrates 10.5 g Sugar 4.1 g Protein 3.4 g Cholesterol 0 mg

48. <u>Crispy Cauliflower & Almonds</u>

Preparation Time: 10 minutes

Cooking Time: 15 minutes

Servings: 4

Ingredients:

- 3 cups cauliflower florets
- 1 tsp garlic, minced
- 1/2 tsp dried thyme
- 1/4 cup breadcrumbs
- 1/4 cup almonds, chopped
- 1/4 cup parmesan cheese, shredded
- 3 tsp olive oil
- Pepper
- Salt

Directions:

1. Line multi-level air fryer basket with parchment paper.
2. In a bowl, toss cauliflower florets with oil, garlic, pepper, and salt.
3. Add cauliflower florets into the multi-level air fryer basket.

4. Place basket into the pot. Secure pot with air fryer lid and cook on air fry mode at 360 F for 10 minutes.

5. Transfer cauliflower florets into the mixing bowl. Add thyme, breadcrumbs, almonds, and cheese and toss until well coated.

6. Return cauliflower mixture into the multi-level air fryer basket.

7. Place basket into the pot. Secure pot with air fryer lid and cook on air fry mode at 360 F for 5 minutes more.

8. Serve and enjoy.

Nutrition: Calories 129 Fat 8.1 g Carbohydrates 10.6 g Sugar 2.5 g Protein 5.5 g Cholesterol 4 mg

49. <u>Cauliflower Roast with Pepperoncini</u>

Preparation Time: 10 minutes

Cooking Time: 15 minutes

Servings: 2

Ingredients:

- 2 cups cauliflower florets
- 1/4 tbsp vinegar
- 2 tbsp almonds, sliced & toasted
- 4 oz jar pepperoncini, drained & chopped
- 1/2 tbsp olive oil
- Pepper
- Salt

Directions:

1. Toss cauliflower florets with oil, pepper, and salt.
2. Add cauliflower florets into the multi-level air fryer basket.
3. Place basket into the pot. Secure pot with air fryer lid and cook on roast mode at 400 F for 15 minutes.
4. Transfer roasted cauliflower florets into the bowl. Add vinegar, almonds, and pepperoncini and toss well.
5. Serve and enjoy.

Nutrition: Calories 100 Fat 6.6 g Carbohydrates 8.6 g Sugar 2.7 g Protein 3.3 g Cholesterol 0 mg

50. Crispy Rosemary Potatoes

Preparation Time: 10 minutes

Cooking Time: 15 minutes

Servings: 4

Ingredients:

- 4 cups baby potatoes, quartered
- 1/2 tsp garlic powder
- 1 tbsp fresh rosemary, chopped
- 1 tbsp olive oil
- 1/4 tsp pepper
- 1/2 tsp salt

Directions:

1. Add potatoes and remaining ingredients into the mixing bowl and toss well.
2. Add potatoes into the multi-level air fryer basket.
3. Place basket into the pot. Secure pot with air fryer lid and cook on air fry mode at 400 F for 15 minutes.
4. Serve and enjoy.

Nutrition: Calories 56 Fat 3.7 g Carbohydrates 5.6 g Sugar 0.1 g Protein 1.1 g Cholesterol 0 mg

Ketogenic Air Fryer Cookbook for Beginners

The complete Keto air fryer cookbook, eat amazing no-fuss dishes with your friends and family

James Ball

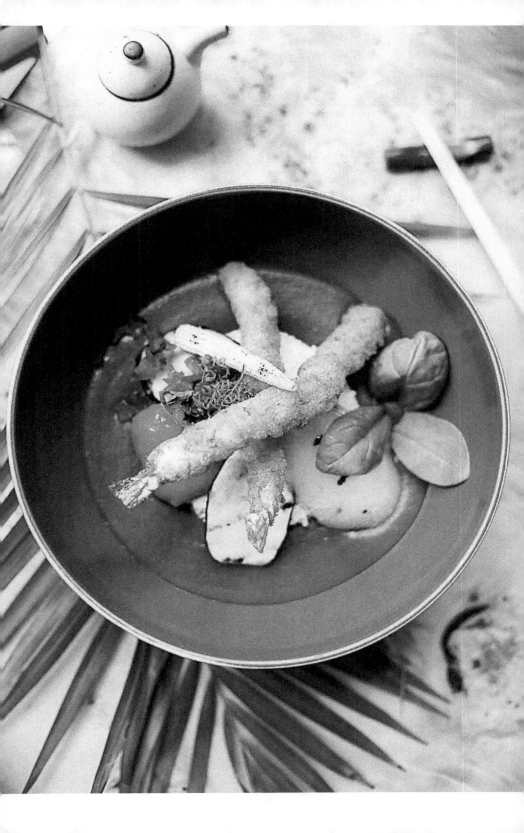

51. Thai Sweet Chili Garlic Shrimp

Basic Recipe

Preparation Time: 10 minutes

Cooking Time: 10 minutes

Servings: 4

Ingredients:

- For shrimp:
- 1 egg
- 12-15 medium shrimps (with shells)
- 30g of tapioca flour
- Ingredients for sauce:
- 1 tablespoon of olive oil
- 1 tablespoon of garlic
- 3 tablespoons of Thai sweet chili sauce
- 2 tablespoons of lime juice
- 2 teaspoons of brown sugar
- 1 teaspoons of chili pepper
- 2 teaspoons of cilantro

Directions:

1. First, you should line your air fryer basket with a sheet of lightly greased aluminum foil.

2. Beat the egg until fully mixed, dip the shrimps into the egg, then dip them into the tapioca flour ensuring that they are evenly covered. Place into the air fryer basket. Spray with cooking oil and cook at 380 degrees Fahrenheit for 6 to 7 minutes, flipping once in the middle. Remove once fully cooked through.

3. Whilst the shrimps are cooking, mince the garlic and add to a wok with olive oil for about one minute until softened. Add the Thai sweet chili sauce, lime juice, brown sugar and chili pepper and stir until the sauce has thickened. Once the shrimps are cooked, add to the sauce and coat.

4. Garnish the shrimps with the cilantro to serve.

Nutrition: Calories 129 Fat 5g Carbs 16g Protein 5g

52. Thai Red Curry Tofu and Potatoes

Basic Recipe

Preparation Time: 10 minutes

Cooking Time: 45 minutes

Servings: 4

Ingredients:

- 1 onion
- ½ tablespoon of olive oil
- 2 tablespoons of lime juice & zest
- 400ml of coconut milk
- 2 tablespoons of red curry
- 2 tablespoons of fish sauce
- 1 tablespoon of brown sugar
- 2 tablespoons of fresh mint
- 2 tablespoons of fresh Basel
- 1 teaspoon of Thai peppers
- 226g of small potatoes
- 1 teaspoon of coarse sea salt
- 1 teaspoon of sea salt
- 1 teaspoon of red curry
- Olive oil spray

- 400g of tofu
- 1 teaspoon of red curry

Directions:

1. First spray the potatoes with cooking oil, sprinkle 1 teaspoon of salt and 1 teaspoon of red curry over the potatoes. Place into the Air Fryer basket and cook for 7 minutes at 400 degrees Fahrenheit. After 7 minutes toss the potatoes around and cook for a further 7 minutes Once the potatoes are crispy you can set them aside.

2. Dry out your tofu by placing paper towels on top and underneath. Use something heavy to press down the tofu and leave to Dry out for 10 minutes Cut your tofu into bite-size pieces. Cover the tofu in 1 teaspoon of red curry. Place the tofu into your Air Fryer, set the temperature to 360 degrees Fahrenheit and cook for 8 minutes Toss around in the basket and cook for an additional 8 minutes

3. To make the sauce, you need to chop the onion into small squares, as well as chopping your basil and mint. Next, you need to heat ½ a tablespoon of oil into a pan, add the onions and cook until translucent. Add

the coconut milk and bring to a boil, stir in the curry, fish sauce and brown sugar. Add the potatoes to the pan and simmer for 10 to 15 minutes

4. Add the lime juice, lime zest and tofu to the mixture, making sure to stir in well. Add the mint and basil and again stir into the mixture. Season it to taste.

Nutrition: Calories 341 Fat 25g Carbs 22g Protein 11g

53. Indian Cauliflower Curry

Basic Recipe

Preparation Time: 5 minutes

Cooking Time: 15 minutes

Servings: 4

Ingredients:

- 240ml of vegetable stock
- 180ml of light coconut milk
- 1 ½ teaspoon of garam masala
- 1 teaspoon of mild curry powder
- 1 teaspoon of garlic puree
- 1/3 teaspoon of turmeric
- ¼ teaspoon of salt
- 350g of cauliflower florets
- 200g of sweet corn kernels
- 3 scallions

Directions:

1. Preheat your Air Fryer to 375 degrees Fahrenheit.
2. Mix the vegetable stock, light coconut milk, garam masala, mild curry powder, garlic puree, turmeric and salt in a large bowl.

3. Add in the cauliflower, sweet corn and the scallions. Mix them in until coated.

4. Place in a dish and put inside the Air Fryer, cook at 375 degrees Fahrenheit for 12 to 15 minutes

Nutrition: Calories 166 Fat 4g Carbs 29g Protein 4g

54. Thai Green Curry Noodles

Intermediate Recipe

Preparation Time: 1 hour and 15 minutes

Cooking Time: 20 minutes

Servings: 6

Ingredients:

- 1kg of shirataki noodles
- 6 tablespoons of soy sauce
- 1 ½ tablespoon of fish sauce
- 1 teaspoon of sesame oil
- ½ teaspoon garlic powder
- 350g of tofu
- 150g of snow peas
- 1 red pepper
- 1 green pepper
- 100g of mushrooms
- 150g of water chestnuts
- 1 teaspoon of coriander paste
- 3 tablespoons of lime juice
- 2 teaspoons of lemongrass paste
- 4 tablespoons of rice wine vinegar

- 350g of napa cabbage

- 2 medium carrots

- 4 green onions

- 6 tablespoons of Thai green curry paste

Directions

1. Firstly, to prepare the vegetables make sure both peppers, mushrooms water chestnuts are sliced thinly. The carrots and cabbage need to be shredded and lastly, the green onions chopped finely. Set aside for later.

2. Place the noodles in a large bowl with 500 ml of boiling water, stirring in 1 tablespoon of the soy sauce. Set aside.

3. Mix 3 tablespoons of the soy sauce, fish sauce, sesame oil and garlic powder together to make a marinade.

4. Cut the tofu into bite-size cubes and put into the marinade, making sure to mix together. Set aside.

5. In a bowl to make the stir-fry veg, mix the snow peas, peppers, mushrooms and water chestnuts. Set aside.

6. To make the dressing, mix the coriander paste, lime juice, lemongrass paste and 4 tablespoons of the Thai green curry paste and 2 tablespoons of the rice vinegar. Set aside.

7. To make the veg base, mix the shredded cabbage, shredded carrots and the chopped green onion. Set aside.

8. Set the Air Fryer temperature to 360 degrees Fahrenheit and spray the basket with cooking oil.

9. Remove the tofu from the marinade and place into the Air Fryer basket, cook for 12 to 13 minutes Make sure to turn halfway through the cooking process. Once done, set aside with a plate on top to keep them warm.

10. Mix the leftover marinade, 2 tablespoons of rice vinegar, 2 tablespoons of soy sauce, 2 tablespoons of the Thai green curry paste, place into a bowl suitable for the Air Fryer, mix in the stir-fry veg and spray with the cooking oil. Cook for 5 minutes

11. Dry out the noodles.

12. In a large bowl, put in: the noodles, the dressing, the tofu cubes, the stir-fry veg and the veg base. Toss with tongs to mix everything together.

Nutrition: Calories 183 Fat 6.1g Carbs 22.7g Protein 9.9g

55. Italian Salmon

Basic Recipe

Preparation Time: 5 minutes

Cooking Time: 10 minutes

Servings: 2

Ingredients:

- 340g of salmon fillets
- 1 ½ tablespoons of butter
- 2 garlic cloves
- 1 tablespoon of lemon juice
- 2 teaspoons of brown sugar
- 2 teaspoons of parsley
- ½ teaspoon of dried Italian seasoning
- ½ teaspoon of pepper
- ½ teaspoon of salt

Directions:

1. To prep, mince the garlic and finely chop the parsley.
2. Melt the butter and mix in the garlic, lemon juice, brown sugar, parsley and Italian seasoning.
3. Coat the salmon fillets in the butter mixture.
4. Next, season the salmon fillets with salt and pepper.

5. Place the salmon fillets in the Air Fryer and cook at 390 degrees Fahrenheit for 7 to 8 minutes Turn halfway through cooking. The internal temperature should be at least 145 degrees Fahrenheit.

Nutrition: Calories 332 Fat 19g Carbs 4g Protein 34g

56. Mexican Taco Salad Bowl

Basic Recipe

Preparation Time: 2 minutes

Cooking Time: 10 minutes

Servings: 2

Ingredients:

- 1 Burrito Sized Flour Tortilla
- Cooking Spray

Directions:

1. Spray both sides of the tortilla with cooking spray.
2. Fold a piece of foil, which is double the size of the tortilla and place it over the tortilla wrap.
3. Place into the Air Fryer and put a bowl just slightly smaller inside, this will help to weigh it down.
4. Cook the tortilla at 400 degrees Fahrenheit for 5 minutes
5. Remove the bowl and then Air Fry for a further 2 minutes
6. Fill the burrito bowl with salad ingredients of your choice.

Nutrition: Calories 220 Fat 20g Carbs 84g Protein 21g

57. Italian Ratatouille

Intermediate Recipe

Preparation Time: 25 minutes

Cooking Time: 25 minutes

Servings: 4

Ingredients:

- ½ Small eggplants
- 1 zucchini
- 1 medium tomato
- ½ large yellow bell pepper
- ½ large red bell peppers
- ½ onions
- 1 cayenne pepper
- 5 basil sprigs
- 2 oregano sprigs
- 1 garlic clove
- ½ teaspoon of salt
- ½ teaspoon of pepper
- 1 tablespoon of olive oil
- 1 tablespoon of white wine
- 1 teaspoon of vinegar

Directions:

1. Preheat your Air Fryer to 400 degrees Fahrenheit.

2. Next, cut the zucchini, tomato, both bell peppers, onion, cayenne pepper into cubes. Then steam and chop the basil and oregano leaves.

3. Mix the eggplant, zucchini, tomato, bell peppers, onions, cayenne pepper, basil, oregano, garlic, salt and pepper in a bowl. Drizzle with the mixture in oil, wine and vinegar.

4. Find a baking dish that fits inside of your Air Fryer and pour the vegetable mixture into the bowl.

5. Put the baking dish into the Air Fryer and cook for 8 minutes Once the 8 minutes are up, stir and then cook for a further 8 minutes Stir again and keep cooking until the vegetables become tender, make sure to stir every 5 minutes for another 10 minutes

Nutrition: Calories 79 Calories Fat 3.8g Carbs 10.2g Protein 2.1g

58. Chinese Crispy Vegetables

Basic Recipe

Preparation Time: 10 minutes

Cooking Time: 15 minutes

Servings: 2

Ingredients:

- 260g of mixed vegetables e.g., Bell peppers, cauliflower, mushrooms, zucchini, baby corn
- 20g of corn-starch
- 20g of all-purpose flour
- ½ teaspoon of garlic powder
- ½ teaspoon of red chili powder
- ½ teaspoon of black pepper powder
- 1 teaspoon of salt
- 1 teaspoon of olive oil
- 2 tablespoons of soy sauce
- 1 tablespoon of chili sauce
- 1 tablespoon of ketchup
- 1 tablespoon of vinegar
- 1 teaspoon of brown sugar
- 1 tablespoon of sesame oil

- 1 teaspoon of sesame seeds

Directions:

1. Cut the cauliflower in small florets. Cube the bell peppers, cut the mushrooms in half. Cut the carrots and zucchini in circles.
2. To make the batter, mix the all-purpose flour, cornstarch, garlic powder, bell pepper powder, red chili powder and the salt together.
3. Add a teaspoon of oil to the batter, mix until not lumpy.
4. Add the vegetables to the batter and make sure they are evenly coated.
5. Preheat your Air Fryer to 350 degrees Fahrenheit.
6. Add the vegetables to the Air Fryer basket and cook for 10 minutes
7. In a saucepan, add a tablespoon of oil, finely chopped garlic, heat until it gives an aroma. Then add the soy sauce, chili sauce, tomato ketchup, vinegar, brown sugar and the black pepper powder.
8. Cook the sauce for a minute then add the Air Fried vegetables and mix well. Make sure the vegetables are evenly coated.

9. Sprinkle the sesame seeds and sesame oil over the vegetables.

Nutrition: Calories 236 Fat 10.5g Carbs 32.2g Protein 4.6g

59. Chinese Salt and Pepper Tofu

Basic Recipe

Preparation Time: 20 minutes

Cooking Time: 15 minutes

Servings: 2

Ingredients:

- 450g of tofu
- ¾ teaspoon of sea salt
- ¾ teaspoon of ground white pepper
- 2 pinches of Chinese spice powder
- 1 teaspoon of sugar
- 3 tablespoons of canola
- 1 tablespoon of corn-starch
- 3 ½ tablespoons of rice flour
- 3 garlic cloves
- 1 serrano chile
- 2 large scallions

Directions:

1. Preheat your Air Fryer to 375 degrees Fahrenheit.

2. Cut tofu into bite-size pieces and mix with ¼ teaspoon of the salt. Put on paper towels and let the moisture Dry out.

3. In a bowl, stir together ¼ teaspoon of salt, 1/8 teaspoon of pepper, Chinese spice and the sugar. Put half of the mixture into a bowl and add the corn-starch and rice flour.

4. Coat the tofu in 1 tablespoon of the canola oil and then cover in the seasoned starch and flour mixture.

5. Put the tofu into the Air Fryer basket and cook at 375 degrees Fahrenheit for 15 minutes Make sure to toss halfway through the cooking process.

6. Whilst cooking, in wok mix 2 tablespoons canola oil, garlic, chili and scallions. Cook for about half a minute until fragrant.

7. Add the tofu to the wok and then sprinkle in the remaining salt, pepper, Chinese spice and sugar mixture. Cook for 1 to 2 minutes, making sure to stir continuously.

Nutrition: Calories 466 Fat 30.9g Carbs 31.6g Protein 21.5g

60. Indian Almond Crusted Fried Masala Fish

Intermediate Recipe

Preparation Time: 30 minutes

Cooking Time: 20 minutes

Servings: 4

Ingredients:

- 900g of fish fillet
- 4 tablespoons of extra virgin olive oil
- ¾ teaspoon of turmeric
- 1 teaspoon of cayenne pepper
- 1 teaspoon of salt
- 1 tablespoon of fenugreek leaves
- 1 ½ teaspoons of ground cumin
- 2 teaspoons of amchoor powder
- 2 tablespoons of ground almonds

Directions:

1. In a bowl, combine the oil, turmeric, cayenne, salt, fenugreek leaves, cumin and amchoor powder. After combining mix in the ground almonds, put the fish

into a bowl and pour the mixture over the fish. Mix around to evenly cover the fish.

2. Put the fish into the Air Fryer basket and cook for 450 degrees Fahrenheit for 10 minutes Turnover and then cook for a further 10 minutes

Nutrition Calories 675 Calories Fat 43.6g Carbs 41.7g Protein 34.5g

61. Sesame Seeds Coated Fish

Basic Recipe

Preparation Time: 20 minutes

Cooking Time: 20 minutes

Servings: 28

Ingredients:

- ½ cup sesame seeds, toasted
- ½ teaspoon dried rosemary, crushed
- 8 tablespoons olive oil
- 14 frozen fish fillets (white fish of your choice)
- 6 eggs
- ½ cup breadcrumbs
- 8 tablespoons plain flour
- Salt and freshly ground black pepper, to taste

Directions:

1. Take three dishes, place flour in one, crack eggs in the other and mix remaining ingredients except fillets in the third one.

2. Now, coat fillets in the flour and dip in the beaten eggs.
3. Then, dredge generously with the sesame seeds mixture.
4. Meanwhile, preheat the air fryer to 390 degrees F and line the air fryer basket with the foil.
5. Arrange fillets in the basket and cook for about 14 minutes, flipping once in the middle way.
6. Take out and serve hot.

Nutrition: Calories 179 Fat 9.3g Carbs: 15.8g Protein 7.7g

62. **Parsley Catfish**

Basic Recipe

Preparation Time: 10 minutes

Cooking Time: 25 minutes

Servings: 4

Ingredients:

- 4 catfish fillets
- 1/4 cup Louisiana Fish fry
- 1 tablespoon olive oil
- 1 tablespoon chopped parsley optional
- 1 lemon, sliced
- Fresh herbs, to garnish

Directions:

1. Preheat air fryer to 400 degrees F.
2. Rinse the fish fillets and pat them try.
3. Rub the fillets with the seasoning and coat well.
4. Spray oil on top of each fillet.
5. Place the fillets in the air fryer basket.
6. Cover the lid and cook for 10 minutes
7. Flip the fillets and cook more for another 10 minutes
8. Flip the fish and cook for 3 minutes until crispy.

9. Garnish with parsley, fresh herbs, and lemon. Serve warm.

Nutrition: Calories 248 Fat 15.7 g Carbs 0.4 g Protein 24.9 g

63. **Seasoned Salmon**

Basic Recipe

Preparation Time: 5 minutes

Cooking Time: 10 minutes

Servings: 4

Ingredients:

- 2 wild caught salmon fillets, 1-1/12-inches thick
- 2 teaspoons avocado oil or olive oil
- 2 teaspoons paprika
- Salt and coarse, to taste
- Black pepper, to taste
- Green herbs, to garnish

Directions:

1. Clean the salmon and let it rest for 1 hour at room temperature.
2. Season the fish with olive oil, salt, pepper, and paprika.
3. Arrange the fish in the air fryer basket.
4. Cook for 7 minutes at 390 degrees.
5. Once done, remove the fish from the fryer.
6. Garnish with fresh herbs.

7. Serve warm.

Nutrition: Calories 249 Fat 11.9 g Carbs 1.8 g Protein 35 g

64. Ranch Fish Fillets

Basic Recipe

Preparation Time: 5 minutes

Cooking Time: 13 minutes

Servings: 4

Ingredients:

- 3/4 cup breadcrumbs or Panko or crushed cornflakes
- 1 packet dry ranch-style dressing mix
- 2 1/2 tablespoons vegetable oil
- 2 eggs beaten
- 4 tilapia salmon or other fish fillets
- Herbs and chilies to garnish

Directions:

1. Preheat the air fryer to 180 degrees F.
2. Mix ranch dressing with panko in a bowl.
3. Whisk eggs in a shallow bowl.
4. Dip each fish fillet in the egg then coat evenly with the panko mixture.
5. Place the fillets in the air fryer.
6. Cook for 13 minutes
7. Serve warm with herbs and chilies.

Nutrition: Calories 301 Fat 12.2 g Carbs: 15 g Protein 28.8 g

65. Crispy Salt and Pepper Tofu

Basic Recipe

Preparation Time: 5 minutes

Cooking Time: 20 minutes

Servings: 4

Ingredients:

- ¼ cup chickpea flour
- ¼ cup arrowroot (or cornstarch)
- 1 teaspoon sea salt
- 1 teaspoon granulated garlic
- ½ teaspoon freshly grated black pepper
- 1 (15-ounce) package tofu, firm or extra-firm
- Cooking oil spray (sunflower, safflower, or refined coconut)
- Asian Spicy Sweet Sauce, optional

Directions:

1. In a medium bowl, combine the flour, arrowroot, salt, garlic, and pepper. Stir well to combine. Cut the tofu into cubes (no need to press—if it's a bit watery, that's fine!). Place the cubes into the flour mixture. Toss well

to coat. Spray the tofu with oil and toss again. (The spray will help the coating better stick to the tofu.)

2. Spray the air fryer basket with the oil. Place the tofu in a single layer in the air fryer basket (you may have to do this in 2 batches, depending on the size of your appliance) and spray the tops with oil. Fry for 8 minutes Remove the air fryer basket and spray again with oil. Toss gently or turn the pieces over. Spray with oil again and fry for another 7 minutes, or until golden-browned and very crisp. Serve immediately, either plain or with the Asian Spicy Sweet Sauce.

Nutrition: Calories 148 Fat 5g Carbs 14g Protein 11g

66. Beef with Beans

Preparation time: 10 minutes

Cooking time: 13 minutes

Servings: 8

Ingredients:

- 12 oz. lean steak
- 1 onion, sliced
- 1 can chopped tomatoes
- 3/4 cup beef stock
- 4 tsp fresh thyme, chopped
- 1 can red kidney beans
- Salt and pepper to taste
- Oven safe bowl

Directions:

1. Preparing the ingredients. Preheat the instant crisp air fryer to 390 degrees.

2. Trim the fat from the meat and cut into thin 1cm strips

3. Add onion slices to the oven safe bowl and place in the instant crisp air fryer.

4. Air frying. Close air fryer lid. Cook for 3 minutes. Add the meat and continue cooking for 5 minutes.

5. Add the tomatoes and their juice, beef stock, thyme and the beans and cook for an additional 5 minutes

6. Season with black pepper to taste.

Nutrition: Calories 98 Fat 7 g Carbohydrates 6 g Sugar 0.4 g Protein 11.8 g Cholesterol 33 mg

67. Easy Pork Roast

Preparation Time: 10 minutes

Cooking Time: 8 hours

Serving: 6

Ingredients:

- 3 lbs. pork shoulder roast, boneless and cut into 4 pieces
- 1/2 tbsp cumin
- 1 tbsp fresh oregano
- 1 cup of grapefruit juice
- Pepper
- Salt

Directions:

1. Season meat with pepper and salt and place into the inner pot of air fryer .
2. Add oregano, cumin, and grapefruit juice into the blender and blend until smooth.
3. Pour blended mixture over meat.
4. Seal the pot with pressure cooking lid and select slow cook mode and cook on low for 8 hours.
5. Remove meat from pot and shred using a fork.

6. Return shredded meat into the pot and stir well.

7. Serve and enjoy.

Nutrition: Calories 599 Fat 46.4 g Carbohydrates 3.8 g Sugar 2.7 g Protein 38.5 g Cholesterol 161 mg

68. Ranch Pork Chops

Preparation Time: 10 minutes

Cooking Time: 30 minutes

Serving: 6

Ingredients:

- 6 pork chops, boneless
- 1/4 cup olive oil
- 1 tsp dried parsley
- 2 tbsp ranch seasoning
- Pepper
- Salt

Directions:

1. Line instant pot air fryer basket with parchment paper.
2. Season pork chops with pepper and salt and place on parchment paper into the air fryer basket.
3. Mix together olive oil, parsley, and ranch seasoning.
4. Spoon oil mixture over pork chops.
5. Place air fryer basket in the pot.
6. Seal the pot with air fryer basket and select bake mode and cook at 400 F for 30 minutes.
7. Serve and enjoy.

Nutrition: Calories 338 Fat 28.3 g Carbohydrates 0 g Sugar 0 g Protein 18 g Cholesterol 69 mg

69. Pork Carnitas

Preparation Time: 10 minutes

Cooking Time: 9 hours

Serving: 6

Ingredients:

- 3 lbs. pork shoulder
- 3 tsp cumin
- 2 orange juice
- 1/2 cup water
- 2 tsp olive oil
- 2 tsp ground coriander
- 2 tsp salt

Directions:

1. Place the pork shoulder into the inner pot of air fryer .
2. Pour remaining ingredients over the pork shoulder.
3. Seal the pot with pressure cooking lid and select slow cooker mode and cook on low for 9 hours.
4. Remove meat from pot and shred using a fork.
5. Serve and enjoy.

Nutrition: Calories 693 Fat 50.4 g Carbohydrates 3.4 g Sugar 2.4 g Protein 53.2 g Cholesterol 204 mg

70. **Pulled Pork**

Preparation Time: 10 minutes

Cooking Time: 50 minutes

Serving: 6

Ingredients:

- 3 lbs. pork butt, cut into large chunks
- 1/2 tsp cumin
- 2 tbsp paprika
- 1 tbsp olive oil
- 1/2 cup water
- 1/2 tsp cayenne pepper
- 1 tbsp oregano
- 1 tsp pepper
- 2 tsp salt

Directions:

1. Add the meat into the inner pot of air fryer and top with olive oil.
2. In a small bowl, mix together paprika, cayenne, oregano, cumin, pepper, and salt and sprinkle over meat.
3. Add water and stir well.

4. Seal the pot with pressure cooking lid and cook on high for 40 minutes.
5. Once done, allow to release pressure naturally for 10 minutes then release remaining pressure using a quick release. Remove lid.
6. Remove meat from pot and shred using a fork.
7. Return shredded meat to the pot and cook on sauté mode for 10 minutes.
8. Stir and serve.

Nutrition: Calories 469 Fat 17.9 g Carbohydrates 2.2 g Sugar 0.3 g Protein 71.1 g Cholesterol 209 mg

71. **Pork Patties**

Preparation Time: 10 minutes

Cooking Time: 15 minutes

Serving: 6

Ingredients:

- 2 lbs. ground pork
- 1 tsp red pepper flakes
- 1 tbsp dried parsley
- 1 1/2 tbsp Italian seasoning
- 1 tsp fennel seed
- 1 tsp paprika
- 2 tbsp olive oil
- 2 tsp salt

Directions:

1. Line instant pot air fryer basket with parchment paper.
2. In a large bowl, mix together ground pork, fennel seed, paprika, red pepper flakes, parsley, Italian seasoning, olive oil, pepper, and salt.
3. Make small patties from meat mixture and place on place on parchment paper into the air fryer basket.
4. Place basket into the pot.

5. Seal the pot with air fryer basket and select bake mode and cook at 375 F for 15 minutes.

6. Serve and enjoy.

Nutrition: Calories 270 Fat 11.2 g Carbohydrates 1 g Sugar 0.4 g Protein 39.7 g Cholesterol 113 mg

72. Herb Pork Tenderloin

Preparation Time: 10 minutes

Cooking Time: 30 minutes

Serving: 4

Ingredients:

- 1 lb. pork tenderloin
- 1 tsp oregano, dried
- 1 tsp thyme, dried
- 1 tsp olive oil
- 1/2 tsp onion powder
- 1/2 tsp garlic powder
- 1/2 tsp pepper
- 1/2 tsp salt

Directions:

1. In a small bowl, mix together onion powder, garlic powder, oregano, thyme, pepper and salt.
2. Coat pork with oil then rub with herb mixture and place into the instant pot air fryer basket.
3. Place basket in the pot.
4. Seal the pot with air fryer lid and select roast mode and cook at 400 F for 30 minutes.

5. Slice and serve.

Nutrition: Calories 177 Fat 5.2 g Carbohydrates 1.1 g Sugar 0.2 g Protein 29.9 g Cholesterol 83 mg

73. <u>Teriyaki Pork</u>

Preparation time: 10 minutes

Cooking time: 40 minutes

Servings: 4

Ingredients:

- 2 lb. pork loin
- 1/2 tsp onion powder
- 1 tsp ground ginger
- 2 tbsp brown sugar
- 1/2 cup water
- 1/4 cup soy sauce
- 1 cup chicken stock
- 1 1/2 tbsp honey
- 2 garlic cloves, crushed

Directions:

1. In a small bowl, mix together all ingredients except meat and stock.
2. Pour the stock into the instant pot.
3. Place meat into the pot then pour bowl mixture over the pork.

4. Seal pot with lid and cook on manual high pressure for 45 minutes.

5. Once done then allow to release pressure naturally then open the lid.

6. Serve and enjoy.

Nutrition: Calories 606 Fat 31.8 g Carbohydrates 13.4 g Sugar 11.4 g Protein 63.3 g Cholesterol 181 mg

74. Easy & Tasty Ribs

Preparation time: 10 minutes

Cooking time: 40 minutes

Servings: 4

Ingredients:

- 2 3/4 lbs. country-style pork ribs
- Dry rub:
- 1 tsp garlic powder
- 1 tbsp brown sugar
- 1 tsp cumin
- 1 tsp pepper
- 1 cup chicken stock
- 1 tsp cayenne pepper
- 1 tsp paprika
- 1 tsp onion powder
- 1 tsp salt

Directions:

1. In a small bowl, mix together all rub ingredients and rub over meat.
2. Pour the stock into the instant pot then place ribs into the pot.

3. Seal pot with lid and cook on high pressure for 45 minutes.

4. Once done then allow to release pressure naturally then open the lid.

5. Stir and serve.

Nutrition: Calories 601 Fat 36.3 g Carbohydrates 4.5 g Sugar 2.9 g Protein 61.3 g Cholesterol 235 mg

75. Air Fryer Steak

Preparation:10 minutes

Cooking time: 35minutes

Servings: 4

Ingredients:

- 2 pounds bone-in-ribeye
- 4 tablespoon butter, softened
- 2 garlic cloves, minced
- 2 teaspoon parsley, freshly chopped
- 1 teaspoon chives, freshly chopped
- 1 teaspoon thyme, freshly chopped
- 1 teaspoon rosemary, freshly chopped
- ½ teaspoon black pepper, freshly ground
- 1 teaspoon kosher salt

Directions:

1. Wash and pat dry the ribeye.
2. In a small bowl, mix the butter and herbs thoroughly.
3. In a plastic wrap, place the butter-herb mix in the center and roll it like a log. Close both ends of the wrap to keep it airtight and refrigerate it until it hardens. It will take about 20 minutes to freeze.

4. Rub the salt and pepper over the steak on both sides.

5. Transfer the steak in the air fryer basket and place it in the inner pot of the instant pot air fryer.

6. Close the crisp cover.

7. Under the air fry mode, select the temperature to 400°f and select timer to 14 minutes.

8. Press start to begin the cooking.

9. Halfway through the cooking, open the crisp cover and flip the steak.

10. After flipping, close the crisp cover to resume the cooking.

11. Now take out the refrigerated herb mix and slice it.

12. After cooking, serve on a plate and top it with the herb slice mix.

Nutrition: Calories: 407, total fat: 22.1g, saturated fat: 11.1g, trans fat: 1g, cholesterol: 178mg, sodium: 823mg, total carbs: 1g, dietary fiber: 0g, sugars: 0g, protein: 52g

76. **Parmesan Pork Chops**

Preparation Time: 10 minutes

Cooking Time: 12 minutes

Serving: 4

Ingredients:

- 1 lb. pork chops, boneless
- 1/4 cup parmesan cheese, grated
- 1/3 cup flour
- 1 tsp paprika
- 1/2 tsp onion powder
- 1 tsp creole seasoning
- 1 tsp garlic powder

Directions:

1. Add all ingredients except pork chops into the zip-lock bag.
2. Add pork chops into the bag. Seal bag and shake well.
3. Place the dehydrating tray in a multi-level air fryer basket and place basket in the instant pot.
4. Place pork chops on dehydrating tray.

5. Seal pot with air fryer lid and select air fry mode then set the temperature to 360 F and timer for 12 minutes. Turn pork chops halfway through.

6. Serve and enjoy.

Nutrition: Calories 424 Fat 29.6 g Carbohydrates 9.2 g Sugar 0.4 g Protein 28.6 g Cholesterol 102 mg

77. Crisp & Tasty Pork Chops

Preparation Time: 10 minutes

Cooking Time: 15 minutes

Serving: 4

Ingredients:

- 4 pork chops, boneless
- 1/2 tsp onion powder
- 1 tsp paprika
- 1/4 cup parmesan cheese, grated
- 1 cup pork rind
- 2 eggs, lightly beaten
- 1/2 tsp chili powder
- 1/4 tsp pepper
- 1/2 tsp salt

Directions:

1. Season pork chops with pepper and salt.
2. Add pork rind in food processor and process until crumbs form.
3. Mix together pork rind crumbs and seasoning in a large bowl.
4. Place egg in a separate bowl.

5. Dip pork chops in egg then coat with pork crumb.

6. Place the dehydrating tray in a multi-level air fryer basket and place basket in the instant pot.

7. Place coated pork chops on dehydrating tray.

8. Seal pot with air fryer lid and select air fry mode then set the temperature to 400 F and timer for 15 minutes. Turn pork chops halfway through.

9. Serve and enjoy.

Nutrition: Calories 330 Fat 24.7 g Carbohydrates 1.2 g Sugar 0.4 g Protein 25 g Cholesterol 160 mg

78. Italian Meatloaf Sliders

Preparation Time: 10 minutes

Cooking Time: 10 minutes

Serving: 8

Ingredients:

- 1 lb. ground beef
- 1/4 cup coconut flour
- 1/2 cup almond flour
- 1 garlic clove, minced
- 1/4 cup onion, chopped
- 2 eggs, lightly beaten
- 1/2 tsp dried tarragon
- 1 tsp Italian seasoning
- 1 tbsp Worcestershire sauce
- 1/4 cup ketchup
- 1/4 tsp pepper
- 1/2 tsp sea salt

Directions:

1. Add all ingredients into the mixing bowl and mix until well combined.

2. Make patties from meat mixture and place them on a plate. Place in refrigerator for 10 minutes.

3. Place the dehydrating tray in a multi-level air fryer basket and place basket in the instant pot.

4. Place patties on dehydrating tray.

5. Seal pot with air fryer lid and select air fry mode then set the temperature to 360 F and timer for 10 minutes. Turn patties halfway through.

6. Serve and enjoy.

Nutrition: Calories 191 Fat 8.5 g Carbohydrates 7 g Sugar 2.4 g Protein 20.8 g Cholesterol 92 mg

79. Zaatar Lamb Chops

Preparation Time: 10 minutes

Cooking Time: 10 minutes

Serving: 4

Ingredients:

- 4 lamb loin chops
- 1/2 tbsp Zaatar
- 1 tbsp fresh lemon juice
- 1 tsp olive oil
- 2 garlic cloves, minced
- Pepper
- Salt

Directions:

1. Coat lamb chops with oil and lemon juice and rubs with zaatar, garlic, pepper, and salt.
2. Place the dehydrating tray in a multi-level air fryer basket and place basket in the instant pot.
3. Place lamb chops on dehydrating tray.
4. Seal pot with air fryer lid and select air fry mode then set the temperature to 400 F and timer for 10 minutes. Turn lamb chops halfway through.

5. Serve and enjoy.

Nutrition: Calories 266 Fat 11.2 g Carbohydrates 0.6 g Sugar 0.1 g Protein 38 g Cholesterol 122 mg

80. Tasty Southern Pork Chops

Preparation Time: 10 minutes

Cooking Time: 15 minutes

Serving: 2

Ingredients:

- 2 pork chops, wash and pat dry
- 2 tbsp flour
- 1 1/2 tbsp buttermilk
- 1/2 tsp Montreal chicken seasoning
- Salt

Directions:

1. Season pork chops with pepper and salt.
2. Coat pork chops with buttermilk.
3. Place pork chops in a zip-lock bag with flour and shake well to coat. Marinate pork chops for 30 minutes.
4. Place the dehydrating tray in a multi-level air fryer basket and place basket in the instant pot.
5. Place marinated pork chops on dehydrating tray.
6. Seal pot with air fryer lid and select air fry mode then set the temperature to 380 F and timer for 15 minutes. Turn pork chops halfway through.
7. Serve and enjoy.

Nutrition: Calories 290 Fat 20.1 g Carbohydrates 6.7 g Sugar 0.6 g Protein 19.2 g Cholesterol 69 mg

81. Baked Mushrooms

Preparation Time: 10 minutes

Cooking Time: 20 minutes

Servings: 4

Ingredients:

- 1 lb. shiitake mushrooms, rinsed & pat dry
- 3/4 tsp dried thyme
- 1/2 tsp garlic powder
- 1 tbsp vinegar
- 1/4 cup olive oil
- 1/4 tsp pepper
- 1/2 tsp salt

Directions:

1. Line multi-level air fryer basket with parchment paper.
2. In a mixing bowl, mix oil, vinegar, garlic powder, thyme, pepper, and salt. Add mushrooms and toss well.
3. Transfer mushrooms into the multi-level air fryer basket.

4. Place basket into the pot. Secure pot with air fryer lid and cook on bake mode at 400 F for 20 minutes.

5. Serve and enjoy.

Nutrition: Calories 172 Fat 12.9 g Carbohydrates 16.1 g Sugar 4.2 g Protein 1.9 g Cholesterol 0 mg

82. Crispy Parmesan Brussels Sprouts

Preparation Time: 10 minutes

Cooking Time: 25 minutes

Servings: 4

Ingredients:

- 1 lb. Brussels sprouts, trimmed & cut in half
- 1/2 cup parmesan cheese, grated
- 1/4 cup breadcrumbs
- 1/4 cup olive oil
- 1 1/2 tsp garlic powder
- 1 1/2 tsp pepper
- 1/2 tsp salt

Directions:

1. Line multi-level air fryer basket with parchment paper.
2. Add Brussels sprouts and remaining ingredients into the mixing bowl and toss until well coated.
3. Transfer Brussels sprouts into the multi-level air fryer basket.
4. Place basket into the pot. Secure pot with air fryer lid and cook on bake mode at 400 F for 25 minutes. Flip Brussels sprouts after 20 minutes.

5. Serve and enjoy.

Nutrition: Calories 225 Fat 15.8 g Carbohydrates 16.8 g Sugar 3.1 g Protein 8.7 g Cholesterol 8 mg

83. Bagel Seasoned Brussels Sprouts

Preparation Time: 10 minutes

Cooking Time: 25 minutes

Servings: 4

Ingredients:

- 1 lb. Brussels sprouts
- 3 tbsp everything bagel seasoning
- 1/4 cup parmesan cheese, grated
- 2 tbsp olive oil
- 2 cups of water

Directions:

1. Add water and Brussels sprouts into the pan, cover, and cook for 10 minutes over medium heat.
2. Drain Brussels sprouts and let it cool completely then cut in half.
3. In a mixing bowl, add Brussels sprouts, bagel seasoning, cheese, and oil and toss well.
4. Line multi-level air fryer basket with parchment paper.
5. Transfer Brussels sprouts into the multi-level air fryer basket.
6. Place basket into the pot. Secure pot with air fryer lid and cook on air fry mode at 375 F for 15 minutes.

7. Serve and enjoy.

Nutrition: Calories 147 Fat 8.7 g Carbohydrates 14.8 g Sugar 2.8 g Protein 6.4 g Cholesterol 4 mg

84. <u>Easy Baked Broccoli</u>

Preparation Time: 10 minutes

Cooking Time: 20 minutes

Servings: 3

Ingredients:

- 1 lb. broccoli florets
- 1/4 cup breadcrumbs
- 1/4 cup cheddar cheese, shredded
- 1/4 tsp Italian seasoning
- 1 garlic, minced
- 1 tbsp olive oil
- Pepper
- Salt

Directions:

1. Line multi-level air fryer basket with parchment paper.
2. Toss broccoli florets with Italian seasoning, garlic, oil, pepper, and salt.
3. Add broccoli florets into the multi-level air fryer basket.
4. Place basket into the pot. Secure pot with air fryer lid and cook on air fry mode at 400 F for 15 minutes.

5. Transfer broccoli florets into the mixing bowl and toss with cheese and breadcrumbs.

6. Return broccoli florets into the multi-level air fryer basket.

7. Place basket into the pot. Secure pot with air fryer lid and cook on air fry mode at 400 F for 5 minutes more.

8. Serve and enjoy.

Nutrition: Calories 168 Fat 8.9 g Carbohydrates 17 g Sugar 3.2 g Protein 7.8 g Cholesterol 10 mg

85. Healthy Roasted Vegetables

Preparation Time: 10 minutes

Cooking Time: 40 minutes

Servings: 4

Ingredients:

- 3 potatoes, diced
- 1/4 cup mushrooms, sliced
- 1/2 zucchini, sliced
- 1/2 yellow summer squash, sliced
- 1 carrot, sliced
- 1 tsp Italian seasoning
- 1 tsp garlic, minced
- 2 tbsp olive oil
- 1/4 tsp pepper
- 1/4 tsp salt

Directions:

1. Line multi-level air fryer basket with parchment paper.
2. Add potatoes, mushrooms, zucchini, squash, carrot, Italian seasoning, garlic, oil, pepper, and salt into the mixing bowl and toss well.
3. Add vegetables into the multi-level air fryer basket.

4. Place basket into the pot. Secure pot with air fryer lid and cook on roast mode at 400 F for 40 minutes.

5. Serve and enjoy.

Nutrition: Calories 189 Fat 7.6 g Carbohydrates 28.5 g Sugar 3.5 g Protein 3.5 g Cholesterol 1 mg

86. Cajun Okra Fries

Preparation Time: 10 minutes

Cooking Time: 30 minutes

Servings: 4

Ingredients:

- 15 oz okra, cut the tops & slice lengthwise
- 1/2 tsp garlic powder
- 1/2 tsp paprika
- 1/4 tsp cayenne
- 2 tbsp olive oil
- 1/2 tsp pepper
- 1 tsp kosher salt

Directions:

1. Line multi-level air fryer basket with parchment paper.
2. Add okra, garlic powder, paprika, cayenne, oil, pepper, and salt into the mixing bowl and toss well.
3. Add okra into the multi-level air fryer basket.
4. Place basket into the pot. Secure pot with air fryer lid and cook on roast mode at 375 F for 25-30 minutes.
5. Serve and enjoy.

Nutrition: Calories 105 Fat 7.3 g Carbohydrates 8.5 g Sugar 1.7 g Protein 2.2 g Cholesterol 0 mg

87. Roasted Green Beans & Carrots

Preparation Time: 10 minutes

Cooking Time: 20 minutes

Servings: 4

Ingredients:

- 1/3 lb. green beans, trimmed
- 1/2 lb. carrots, trimmed, peeled & sliced
- 1 tbsp butter
- 1/4 cup honey
- 1 tbsp olive oil
- 1/4 tsp pepper
- 1/4 tsp salt

Directions:

1. Line multi-level air fryer basket with parchment paper.
2. In a bowl, add carrots, green beans, olive oil, pepper, and salt and toss well.
3. Add carrots and green beans into the multi-level air fryer basket.
4. Place basket into the pot. Secure pot with air fryer lid and cook on roast mode at 400 F for 20 minutes.

5. Meanwhile, in a small saucepan add butter and honey and cook over medium heat for 2 minutes.

6. Remove roasted carrots and green beans from pot and place into the mixing bowl. Pour honey-butter mixture over roasted vegetables and toss well to coat.

7. Serve and enjoy.

Nutrition: Calories 155 Fat 6.4 g Carbohydrates 25.8 g Sugar 20.7 g Protein 1.3 g Cholesterol 8 mg

88. Green Beans with Cherry Tomatoes

Preparation Time: 10 minutes

Cooking Time: 20 minutes

Servings: 2

Ingredients:

- 1/2 lb. green beans, trimmed
- 1 cup cherry tomatoes, cut in half
- 1/4 cup parmesan cheese, shredded
- 1/4 cup balsamic vinegar
- 1 tbsp olive oil
- 1/4 tsp pepper
- 1/4 tsp salt

Directions:

1. Line multi-level air fryer basket with parchment paper.
2. In a mixing bowl, add tomatoes, green beans, oil, pepper, and salt and toss well to coat.
3. Add tomatoes and green beans into the multi-level air fryer basket.
4. Place basket into the pot. Secure pot with air fryer lid and cook on roast mode at 400 F for 20 minutes.

5. Meanwhile, in a small saucepan add vinegar and cook until reduced by half.

6. Remove beans and tomatoes from the pot and sprinkle with cheese and drizzle with vinegar.

7. Serve and enjoy.

Nutrition: Calories 154 Fat 9.7 g Carbohydrates 12.4 g Sugar 4.1 g Protein 6.5 g Cholesterol 8 mg

89. Baked Brussels Sprouts & Asparagus

Preparation Time: 10 minutes

Cooking Time: 20 minutes

Servings: 3

Ingredients:

- 1/2 lb. Brussels sprouts, cut in half
- 1/2 lb. asparagus, trimmed
- 2 tbsp parmesan cheese, shredded
- 1/2 tsp garlic powder
- 2 tbsp olive oil
- Pepper
- Salt

Directions:

1. Line multi-level air fryer basket with parchment paper.
2. In a bowl, toss Brussels sprouts, asparagus, garlic powder, oil, pepper, and salt.
3. Add Brussels sprouts and asparagus into the multi-level air fryer basket.
4. Place basket into the pot. Secure pot with air fryer lid and cook on bake mode at 400 F for 20 minutes. Stir after 15 minutes.

5. Sprinkle parmesan cheese on top of baked vegetables and serve.

Nutrition: Calories 129 Fat 10.5 g Carbohydrates 10.3 g Sugar 3.2 g Protein 5.6 g Cholesterol 3 mg

90. Roasted Zucchini, Tomatoes & Squash

Preparation Time: 10 minutes

Cooking Time: 30 minutes

Servings: 3

Ingredients:

- 1/2 lb. zucchini, cut into slices
- 7 oz cherry tomatoes, cut in half
- 1/2 cup parmesan cheese, shredded
- 3/4 tsp Italian seasoning
- 2 garlic cloves, minced
- 1/2 lb. yellow squash, cut slices
- 1 1/2 tbsp olive oil
- Pepper
- Salt

Directions:

1. Line multi-level air fryer basket with parchment paper.
2. In a large bowl, toss zucchini, tomatoes, squash, Italian seasoning, garlic, cheese, oil, pepper, and salt.
3. Add vegetable mixture into the multi-level air fryer basket.

4. Place basket into the pot. Secure pot with air fryer lid and cook on roast mode at 400 F for 30 minutes.

5. Serve and enjoy.

Nutrition: Calories 151 Fat 11 g Carbohydrates 9 g Sugar 4.5 g Protein 7.4 g Cholesterol 12 mg

91. <u>Salmon Crisps</u>

Preparation Time: 5-10 min.

Cooking Time: 12 min

Servings: 2-4

Ingredients:

- 2 tablespoons dill, chopped
- ½ cup panko breadcrumbs
- ¼ teaspoon ground black pepper
- 2 teaspoons mustard, Dijon
- 2 tablespoons of canola mayonnaise
- 2 cans (5 ounces) salmon, unsalted, with bones and skin
- 2 lemon wedges
- 1 egg, large

Directions:

1. In a mixing bowl, add the salmon, dill, panko, mayonnaise, pepper, and mustard. Combine the ingredients to mix well with each other. Prepare cakes from the mixture.

2. Grease Air Fryer Basket with some cooking spray.

3. Place Instant Pot Air Fryer Crisp over kitchen platform. Press Air Fry, set the temperature to 400°F and set the timer to 5 minutes to preheat. Press "Start" and allow it to preheat for 5 minutes.

4. In the inner pot, place the Air Fryer basket. In the basket, add the salmon cakes.

5. Close the Crisp Lid and press the "Bake" setting. Set temperature to 400°F and set the timer to 12 minutes. Press "Start." Flip the cakes halfway down.

6. Open the Crisp Lid after cooking time is over. Serve with your choice of dip or tomato ketchup.

Nutrition: Calories: 287 Fat: 15g Saturated Fat: 3g Trans Fat: 0g Carbohydrates: 16g Fiber: 2g Sodium: 257mg Protein: 26g

92. Wholesome Asparagus

Preparation Time: 5-10 min.

Cooking Time: 10 min.

Number of Servings: 4

Ingredients:

- pound (½ bunch) asparagus, washed and trimmed
- ½ teaspoon Himalayan salt
- 1 olive oil spray
- 1/4 teaspoon garlic powder
- 1 tablespoons sherry vinegar or red-wine vinegar
- 1 teaspoon chili powder or 1/2 teaspoon smoked paprika

Directions:

1. Add the asparagus in the frying basket, coat with the oil spray, add the chili powder/paprika, garlic powder and salt on top. Stir well to coat evenly.

2. Place Instant Pot Air Fryer Crisp over kitchen platform. Press Air Fry, set temperature to 400°F and set timer to 5 minutes to preheat. Press "Start" and allow it to preheat for 5 minutes.

3. In the inner pot, place the Air Fryer basket. In the basket, add the asparagus mixture.

4. Close the Crisp Lid and press "Air Fry" setting. Set temperature to 400°F and set timer to 10 minutes. Press "Start".

5. Half way down, open the Crisp Lid, shake the basket and close the lid to continue cooking for remaining time.

6. Open the Crisp Lid after cooking time is over. Drizzle with the vinegar on top and serve with your choice of dip or ketchup.

Nutrition: Calories: 62 Fat: 4g Saturated Fat: 5g Trans Fat: 0g Carbohydrates: 6g Fiber: 5g Sodium: 277mg Protein: 3g

93. Apple Sweet Chips

Preparation Time: 5-10 min.

Cooking Time: 12 min.

Servings: 2-3

Ingredients:

- 2 teaspoons sugar
- ½ teaspoon ground cinnamon
- 2 large apples, cored and sliced

Directions:

1. In a bowl, mix the apple pieces with sugar and cinnamon. Place Instant Pot Air Fryer Crisp over kitchen platform. Press Air Fry, set the temperature to 400°F and set the timer to 5 minutes to preheat. Press "Start" and allow it to preheat for 5 minutes. In the inner pot, place the Air Fryer basket. In the basket, add the coated apples. Do not overlap. Close the Crisp Lid and press the "Roast" setting. Set temperature to 350°F and set the timer to 12 minutes. Press "Start." Halfway down, open the Crisp Lid, shake the basket and close the lid to continue cooking for the remaining time. Open the Crisp Lid after cooking time is over. Serve warm.

Nutrition: Calories: 132 Fat: 5g Saturated Fat: 0g Trans Fat: 0g Carbohydrates: 35g Fiber: 5g Sodium: 54mg Protein: 1g

94. Creamed Toasted Sticks

Preparation Time: 5-10 min.

Cooking Time: 8 min.

Servings: 5-6

Ingredients:

- 1/3 cup whole milk
- 1/3 cup heavy cream
- 2 large eggs
- 1/4 teaspoon ground cinnamon
- 3 tablespoon granulated sugar
- 6 thick bread slices cut into 3 parts
- 1/2 teaspoon pure vanilla extract
- Kosher salt and maple syrup to taste

Directions:

1. In a mixing bowl, beat the eggs and add the sugar, milk, cinnamon, and salt; combine well. Coat the bread slices with the mixture.

2. Place Instant Pot Air Fryer Crisp over kitchen platform. Press Air Fry, set the temperature to 400°F and set the timer to 5 minutes to preheat. Press "Start" and allow it to preheat for 5 minutes.

3. In the inner pot, place the Air Fryer basket. Line it with a parchment paper, add the bread slices.

4. Close the Crisp Lid and press the "Air Fry" setting. Set temperature to 370°F and set the timer to 8 minutes. Press "Start."

5. Halfway down, open the Crisp Lid, shake the basket and close the lid to continue cooking for the remaining time.

6. Open the Crisp Lid after cooking time is over. Serve warm with the maple syrup on top.

Nutrition: Calories: 146 Fat: 5g Saturated Fat: 1g Trans Fat: 0g Carbohydrates: 5g Fiber: 1g Sodium: 139mg
Protein: 4g

95. <u>Spicy Kale Chips</u>

Preparation Time: 5-10 min.

Cooking Time: 5 min.

Servings: 2-3

Ingredients:

- 1 bunch of Tuscan kale (stems removed and leaves cut into 2-inch pieces)
- 2 tablespoons olive oil
- 1/4 teaspoon crushed red pepper
- 1/4 teaspoon salt
- 1/4 teaspoon paprika
- 1/4 teaspoon garlic powder

Directions:

1. In a mixing bowl, add the olive oil, kale leaves, and spices. Combine the ingredients to mix well with each other.

2. Place Instant Pot Air Fryer Crisp over kitchen platform. Press Air Fry, set the temperature to 400°F and set the timer to 5 minutes to preheat. Press "Start" and allow it to preheat for 5 minutes.

3. In the inner pot, place the Air Fryer basket. In the basket, add the kale mixture.

4. Close the Crisp Lid and press the "Air Fry" setting. Set temperature to 390°F and set the timer to 5 minutes. Press "Start."

5. Halfway down, open the Crisp Lid, shake the basket and close the lid to continue cooking for the remaining time.

6. Open the Crisp Lid after cooking time is over. Season to taste and serve warm.

Nutrition: Calories: 82 Fat: 6g Saturated Fat: 5g Trans Fat: 0g Carbohydrates: 3g Fiber: 5g Sodium: 258mg Protein: 5g

96. <u>Classic French Fries</u>

Preparation Time: 5-10 min.

Cooking Time: 24 min.

Servings: 4

Ingredients: 1-pound sweet potatoes, cut into French Fries size

- ¼ teaspoon garlic powder
- Salt to taste
- Olive oil

Directions:

1. In a mixing bowl, add the olive oil, potatoes, salt, and garlic powder. Combine the ingredients to mix well with each other. Place Instant Pot Air Fryer Crisp over kitchen platform. Press Air Fry, set the temperature to 400°F and set the timer to 5 minutes to preheat. Press "Start" and allow it to preheat for 5 minutes. In the inner pot, place the Air Fryer basket. In the basket, add the potato mixture. Close the Crisp Lid and press the "Air Fry" setting. Set temperature to 380°F and set the timer to 18-20 minutes. Press "Start." Halfway down, open the Crisp Lid, shake the basket and close the lid to continue cooking for the remaining time. Open the

Crisp Lid after cooking time is over. Season to taste and serve warm.

Nutrition: Calories: 156 Fat: 5g Saturated Fat: 1g Trans Fat: 0g Carbohydrates: 22g Fiber: 3g Sodium: 93mg Protein: 5g

97. Crunchy Zucchini Chips

Preparation Time: 5 min.

Cooking Time: 12 min.

Servings: 4

Ingredients:

- 1 medium zucchini, thinly sliced
- 3/4 cup Parmesan cheese, grated
- 1 cup Panko breadcrumbs
- 1 large egg, beaten

Directions:

1. In a mixing bowl, add the Parmesan cheese and panko breadcrumbs. Combine the ingredients to mix well with each other.

2. In a mixing bowl, beat the eggs. Coat the zucchini slices with the eggs and then with the crumb mixture. Spray the slices with some cooking spray.

3. Place Instant Pot Air Fryer Crisp over kitchen platform. Press Air Fry, set the temperature to 400°F and set the timer to 5 minutes to preheat. Press "Start" and allow it to preheat for 5 minutes.

4. In the inner pot, place the Air Fryer basket. Line it with a parchment paper, add the zucchini slices.

5. Close the Crisp Lid and press the "Air Fry" setting. Set temperature to 350°F and set the timer to 10-12 minutes. Press "Start."
6. Halfway down, open the Crisp Lid, shake the basket and close the lid to continue cooking for the remaining time.
7. Open the Crisp Lid after cooking time is over. Serve warm.

Nutrition: Calories: Fat: g Saturated   Fat: g Trans   Fat: 0g Carbohydrates: g Fiber: g Sodium: mg Protein: g

98. <u>Cauliflower Fritters</u>

Preparation Time: 5-10 min.

Cooking Time: 8 min.

Servings: 6-8

Ingredients:

- 1/3 cup shredded mozzarella cheese
- 1/3 cup shredded sharp cheddar cheese
- ½ cup chopped parsley
- 1 cup Italian breadcrumbs
- 3 chopped scallions
- 1 head of cauliflower, cut into florets
- 1 egg
- 2 minced garlic cloves

Directions:

1. Blend the florets into a blender to make the rice like structure. Add in a bowl. Mix in the pepper, salt, egg, cheeses, breadcrumbs, garlic, and scallions. Prepare 15 patties from the mixture. Coat them with some cooking spray.

2. Place Instant Pot Air Fryer Crisp over kitchen platform. Press Air Fry, set the temperature to 400°F

and set the timer to 5 minutes to preheat. Press "Start" and allow it to preheat for 5 minutes.

3. In the inner pot, place the Air Fryer basket. In the basket, add the patties.

4. Close the Crisp Lid and press the "Air Fry" setting. Set temperature to 390°F and set the timer to 8 minutes. Press "Start."

5. Halfway down, open the Crisp Lid, shake the basket and close the lid to continue cooking for the remaining time.

6. Open the Crisp Lid after cooking time is over. Serve warm.

Nutrition: Calories: 235 Fat: 19g Saturated Fat: 8g Trans Fat: 0g Carbohydrates: 31g Fiber: 5g Sodium: 542mg Protein: 6g

99. <u>Lemon Potato Crisp</u>

Preparation Time: 5-10 min.

Cooking Time: 18 min.

Servings: 4

Ingredients:

- 1 teaspoon Cajun seasoning

- ½ teaspoon ground black pepper

- 1 teaspoon Italian seasoning

- 1 teaspoon garlic powder

- 1-pound baby potatoes, unpeeled and halved

- 1 tablespoon virgin olive oil

- 2 lemons, cut into wedges

- 2 teaspoon kosher salt

- ¼ cup finely chopped parsley

Directions:

1. In a mixing bowl, add the garlic powder, halved potatoes, Cajun seasoning, Italian seasoning, kosher salt, and potatoes. Combine the ingredients to mix well with each other.

2. Place Instant Pot Air Fryer Crisp over kitchen platform. Press Air Fry, set the temperature to 400°F

and set the timer to 5 minutes to preheat. Press "Start" and allow it to preheat for 5 minutes.

3. In the inner pot, place the Air Fryer basket. In the basket, add the potatoes.

4. Close the Crisp Lid and press the "Air Fry" setting. Set temperature to 400°F and set the timer to 18 minutes. Press "Start."

5. Halfway down, open the Crisp Lid, shake the basket and close the lid to continue cooking for the remaining time.

6. Open the Crisp Lid after cooking time is over. Serve warm with lemon wedges and parsley on top.

Nutrition: Calories: 159 Fat: 4g Saturated Fat: 1g Trans Fat: 0g Carbohydrates: 22g Fiber: 5g Sodium: 619mg
Protein: 5g

100. Spiced Chickpeas

Preparation Time: 5-10 min.

Cooking Time: 20 min.

Servings: 4

Ingredients:

- 15 ounces canned chickpeas, drained and dried
- 1 teaspoon salt
- ¼ teaspoon cumin powder
- ¼ teaspoon cayenne pepper powder

Directions:

1. Drain the canned chickpeas using a colander. Rinse and drain the water thoroughly. In a bowl, combine the spices.

2. Place Instant Pot Air Fryer Crisp over kitchen platform. Press Air Fry, set the temperature to 400°F and set the timer to 5 minutes to preheat. Press "Start" and allow it to preheat for 5 minutes.

3. In the inner pot, place the Air Fryer basket. In the basket, add the chickpeas.

4. Close the Crisp Lid and press the "Air Fry" setting. Set temperature to 390°F and set the timer to 20 minutes. Press "Start."

5. Halfway down, open the Crisp Lid, sprinkle half the seasoning mix, shake the basket and close the lid to continue cooking for the remaining time.
6. Open the Crisp Lid after cooking time is over. Sprinkle remaining seasoning and combine. Serve warm.

Nutrition: Calories: 186 Fat: 5g Saturated Fat: 5g Trans Fat: 0g Carbohydrates: 24g Fiber: 5g Sodium: 789mg Protein: 8g

CONCLUSION

In this cookbook, we introduced a new member of the Instant Pot family, the Instant Pot Pro Crisp Air Fryer. It uses two different cooking techniques, one for pressure cooking and the other for air frying. The instant pot pro crisp air fryer comes with two lids, one for pressure cooking and another for air frying.

The cookbook contains healthy, delicious and mouth-watering recipes. The book contains all types of recipes starting from breakfast to desserts. The recipes in this cookbook are unique and written with step-by-step instructions. All the recipes are described with their perfect preparation and cooking time. Each recipe ends with their exact nutritional information.